The Impact of PTSD on Psychological Well-being and PTG:

The Role of Trauma Centrality, Emotion Regulation, and Attachment

创伤后应激障碍对心理健康
与创伤后成长的影响：
创伤中心性、情绪调节与依恋的作用

王娜 著

华中科技大学出版社
http://press.hust.edu.cn
中国·武汉

图书在版编目（CIP）数据

创伤后应激障碍对心理健康与创伤后成长的影响：创伤中心性、情绪调节与依恋的作用：

英文／王娜著. -- 武汉：华中科技大学出版社，2024. 10. -- ISBN 978-7-5772-1369-9

Ⅰ. R749；G444

中国国家版本馆 CIP 数据核字第 2024U9H927 号

创伤后应激障碍对心理健康与创伤后成长的影响：

创伤中心性、情绪调节与依恋的作用   王娜 著

The Impact of PTSD on Psychological Well-being and PTG：

The Role of Trauma Centrality, Emotion Regulation, and Attachment

策划编辑：江 畅

责任编辑：姜雯霏   王炳伦

封面设计：王 琛

责任监印：朱 玢

出版发行：华中科技大学出版社（中国·武汉）   电话：(027)81321913

      武汉市东湖新技术开发区华工科技园   邮编：430223

录   排：华中科技大学惠友文印中心

印   刷：武汉科源印刷设计有限公司

开   本：710mm×1000mm   1/16

印   张：12.75

字   数：242 千字

版   次：2024 年 10 月第 1 版第 1 次印刷

定   价：68.00 元

Abstract

It has been widely documented that following a trauma, adolescent victims can experience psychopathologies such as posttraumatic stress disorder (PTSD) alongside psychiatric co-morbid symptoms. However, this is not the case for all adolescents with some youths appearing unaffected, and others even thriving or gaining benefits from their fearful experiences in a phenomenon termed posttraumatic growth (PTG). Nevertheless, the relationship between PTSD and PTG is controversial in the literature.

In addition, trauma can alter self-concept and trigger coping, both of which may in turn shape victims' psychological functioning and posttraumatic adaptation. Thus, it is assumed that alterations in self-concept (trauma centrality) and coping (cognitive emotion regulation, CER) might mediate the impact of PTSD from past trauma on negative and positive psychological outcomes measured as psychiatric co-morbidity and posttraumatic growth. Also, these traumatic responses could be affected by the quality of parental attachment, especially in the context of a poor child-caregiver relationship (unresolved attachment), given the significant role of supportive others in a child's posttraumatic adjustment. All of these, however, have not been clarified among adolescents. Accordingly, the current thesis, composed of four consecutive studies with cross-sectional and longitudinal designs, aimed to address the impact of PTSD from past trauma on psychiatric co-morbidity and posttraumatic growth among Chinese adolescents and elucidate the roles of trauma centrality, cognitive emotion regulation, and unresolved attachment. In addition, as egocentrism is endemic among adolescents and might distort cognitions to affect posttraumatic reactions, it has been adjusted for in the present thesis.

Four independent samples of Chinese adolescents were recruited for the four consecutive studies in the present thesis. Participants were asked to complete self-report questionnaires measuring PTSD, psychiatric co-morbidity, posttraumatic growth, trauma centrality, cognitive emotion regulation, unresolved attachment, and potential confounding factors (i.e., demographic information, academic stress, and egocentrism). Network analysis, structural equation modeling (SEM), and Latent Profile Analysis (LPA) were then adopted to analyze the data. Overall, PTSD was robustly associated with negative and positive psychological outcomes of psychiatric co-morbidity and posttraumatic growth. In addition, whilst trauma centrality mediated the impact of PTSD from past trauma on psychiatric co-morbidity and posttraumatic growth in the cross-sectional study, this was not verified by the subsequent longitudinal investigation. The two types of cognitive emotion regulation (i.e., adaptive CER and maladaptive CER) respectively mediated the effects of PTSD from past trauma on posttraumatic growth but not on psychiatric co-morbidity. The co-existence of PTSD from past trauma, cognitive emotion regulation, and unresolved attachment influenced the development of psychiatric co-morbidity and posttraumatic growth, giving rise to four latent profiles of adolescents who generally differed in the levels of these two outcomes. For example, adolescents in the high trauma group (one of the four profiles) experienced the greatest severity of psychiatric co-morbidity and the lowest level of posttraumatic growth compared to the other three groups.

To conclude, following fearful events, Chinese adolescents could experience both psychological distress and positive changes. Moreover, whilst trauma may change adolescents' self-understanding, the effect of this alteration on the aforesaid psychological outcomes cannot be predicted. Nevertheless, posttraumatic coping, characterized by cognitive emotion regulation, seemed to have a unique impact on positive changes but not on distress. Specifically, the adaptive pattern and maladaptive pattern of cognitive emotion regulation respectively served as a protector and an inflictor for the nurturance of personal growth. In addition, attachment difficulties could co-exist with traumatic experiences and coping to influence the aforementioned positive and negative psychological reactions.

Keywords: posttraumatic stress, co-morbidity, centrality, emotion regulation, attachment, growth

摘　　要

广泛研究表明，经历创伤事件后，青少年受害者可能会产生精神病理反应，如创伤后应激障碍与精神并发症。然而，并非所有的青少年都如此。有些青少年可能并未受影响，另一些人甚至能从创伤经历中受益，这种现象被称为创伤后成长。然而，创伤后成长与创伤后应激障碍之间的关系在文献里颇有争议。

此外，创伤可以改变个体的自我概念，触发应对措施，进而影响受害者的心理功能与创伤后适应。因此，我们认为，自我概念（创伤中心性，trauma centrality）和应对策略（认知情绪调节，cognitive emotion regulation）的改变可能会介导创伤后应激障碍对精神并发症与创伤后成长的影响。考虑到支持者在儿童或青少年创伤后适应中扮演的重要角色，我们提出，精神并发症与创伤后成长还可能受亲子依恋的影响，尤其在亲子关系较差（未解决的依恋，unresolved attachment）的情况下。然而，以上所有假设在青少年群体中都还未得到阐明。因此，本文采用横断面设计和纵向设计，由四项连续研究组成，旨在探讨创伤后应激障碍对中国青少年精神并发症与创伤后成长的影响，并阐明创伤中心性、认知情绪调节和未解决的依恋在其中的作用。此外，由于自我中心主义在青少年中普遍存在，它可能扭曲认知，影响创伤后的心理反应，因此本文将对自我中心主义的影响进行控制调整。

本文的四项连续研究招募了四个独立的中国青少年样本。受试者完成了关于创伤后应激障碍、精神并发症、创伤后成长、创伤中心性、认知情绪调节、未解决的依恋和潜在的混杂因素（如人口统计学变量、学业压力和自我中心主义）的自我报告问卷。数据分析采用了网络分析（network analysis）、结构方程模型（structural equation modeling，SEM）与潜在剖面分析（Latent Profile Analysis，LPA）。总体来说，创伤后应激障碍与精神并发症和创伤后成长密切相关。此外,虽然在横断面调查中,创伤中心性介导了创伤后应激障碍对精神并发症和创伤后成长的影响,但后续的纵向研究没有证实这一发现。两种认知情绪调节(适应性认知情绪调节和不适应性认知情绪调节)分别介导了创伤后应激障碍对创伤后成长的影响,但它们对精神并发症的影响不显著。创伤后应激障碍能与认知情绪调节和未解决的依恋共存,这种共存区分出了四种不同类型的青少年,这四类青少年经历了不同程度的精神并发症与创伤后成长。例如,与其他三组青少年相比,高创伤组的个体表现出最严重的精神并发症与最少的创伤后成长。

总而言之,创伤事件发生后,中国青少年既可能遭受精神痛苦也可能产生积极变化。虽然创伤也会改变青少年的自我概念,但这种改变对上述两种心理结果的影响难以预测。以认知情绪调节为代表的创伤后应对,似乎对积极变化有独特的影响,对精神痛苦却没有影响。具体而言,认知情绪调节的适应模式和不适应模式分别能促进和抑制青少年的个人成长。此外,依恋困难可能与创伤经历和应对方式并存,从而影响上述积极和消极的心理反应。

关键词:创伤后压力、并发症、中心性、情绪调节、依恋、成长

List of Abbreviations

PTSD	Posttraumatic Stress Disorder
GHQ	The General Health Questionnaire
PTG	Posttraumatic Growth
CES	The Centrality of Event Scale
CER	Cognitive Emotion Regulation
ACER	Adaptive Cognitive Emotion Regulation
MCER	Maladaptive Cognitive Emotion Regulation
I/Int	Intrusion
A/Avo	Avoidance
NACM/Neg	Negative Alterations in Cognitions and Mood
AAR/Alt	Alterations in Arousal and Reactivity
Ref	Reference Point
Cen	Central to One's Identity
Tur	Turning Point
So	Somatic Symptoms
An	Anxiety and Insomnia
Sd	Social Dysfunction
De	Severe Depression
RO	Relating to Others
NP	New Possibilities
PS	Personal Strength
SC	Spiritual Change
AL	Appreciation of Life
UA	Unresolved Attachment

Contents

Chapter 1　General Introduction

1.1　Research Background

1.1.1　Past Trauma and Psychological Distress among Adolescents

1.1.1.1　Definition, Types, and Prevalence of Trauma

Originating from Greek, the word "trauma" was initially used in medical situations that involved physical wounds. Afterwards, this term was gradually applied in psychiatry and clinical psychology to signify psychological wounds (Perrotta, 2019). Psychological trauma, despite the widespread controversies over its definition, is generally accepted by trauma researchers as the damage to a victim's mental state resulting from inadequate resolution of one or more devastating events. These events usually generate overwhelming stress beyond the victim's ability to cope, which could go on to threaten psychophysical integrity, alter self-capacities, and produce extremities of impotence and vulnerability (Janet, 1901; Pearlman & Saakvitne, 1995; Sar & Ozturk, 2006). To facilitate the operability of psychological trauma, the DSM-V Criteria A has specified that a traumatic experience should be the exposure to actual or threatened serious injury, actual or threatened death, or actual or threatened sexual violence, and has provided a list of potentially traumatic events concerning, but not limited to, physical or sexual abuse, life-threatening illness or injury, the loss of a close family member, relative, or friend, being hit by natural disasters, and getting hurt in serious accidents (e.g., explosion, plane crash, car accident, and radiation) (American Psychiatric Association, 2013). Also, the DSM-V Criteria A stipulates that the exposure to a traumatic event must happen in one of the following four forms: 1) direct exposure; 2) witnessing in person; 3) learning that the traumatic event happened to someone close; and 4) being repeatedly or intensively exposed to the aversive details of trauma usually on professional duties, for instance, clinical psychiatrists exposed to the details of child abuse cases, emergency workers, and those collecting bodies or body parts (American Psychiatric Association, 2013).

Specific traumatic events could be further classified into several broad types. The current thesis will review two of the most popular taxonomies. Built upon the work of Terr (1991) and expanding on it (Solomon & Heide, 1999), the first approach differentiated three types of trauma with reference to trauma complexity: 1) Type I trauma as a result of being exposed to one single event (e.g., one single blow of a natural disaster or transportation accident, or witnessing serious injury or death), 2) Type II trauma resulting from exposure to multiple events (e.g., multiple blows of repeated physical, sexual, or emotional abuse, or witnessing prolonged domestic violence) (Terr, 1991), and 3) Type III trauma which was expanded on the basis of Type II trauma and referred to repeated exposure to more extreme events that started in early childhood and lasted for years (e.g., multiple severe blows from enduring physical violence by sadistic caregivers or prolonged sexual abuse by multiple perpetrators at an early age of the victim) (Solomon & Heide, 1999). Whilst survivors of Type I trauma reported some levels of PTSD symptoms and detailed memories of the

2

precipitating event, Type Ⅱ trauma was usually associated with poor self-esteem, shame, dependency, moderate PTSD symptoms, and interpersonal trust difficulties (Terr, 1991). Type Ⅲ trauma, the most complex category, was undoubtedly related to the broadest range of and the greatest severity of internalizing and externalizing problems, including high levels of depression, anxiety and PTSD symptoms, dissociation, emotion dysregulation, trust crisis, abnormal eating, and suicidality (Solomon & Heide, 1999).

The other taxonomy categorized traumatic events according to the principles of a) whether the event is in man's control or not, and b) if it is, whether the event is deliberately perpetrated. In this case, three types of trauma could emerge: 1) natural disasters which occur naturally out of man's control (e.g., earthquake, flood, hurricane, and tornado), 2) unintended manmade trauma, an event that is caused by a human but not deliberately (e.g., boat accident, train wreck, and accidental explosion), and 3) intended interpersonal trauma which is deliberately perpetrated by the perpetrator(s) (e.g., physical violence, sexual assault, emotional abuse, captivity, and homicide). Intended interpersonal trauma tends to be associated with greater severities of PTSD and general psychological disorders than natural disasters and unintended manmade trauma (Breslau et al., 1999; Creamer et al., 2001; Kilpatrick et al., 1997). This might be because intended interpersonal trauma could trigger a sense of betrayal (Freyd, 1994) and violate victims' core beliefs and basic assumptions regarding the trustworthiness and benevolence of others (Janoff-Bulman, 1992). This would especially be the case in a child-caregiver relationship when the caregiver was the perpetrator.

Exposure to trauma has proven to be a statistically normal experience by studies focusing on adolescents from China and other countries (van der Kolk, 2005). For example, before entering adulthood, 62%-90% of adolescents from countries other than China can have experienced at least one type of trauma, including child maltreatment, bereavement, a natural hazard, or a transportation accident (McLaughlin et al., 2013; Ghazali et al., 2014; Elklit, 2002; Elklit & Petersen, 2008; Salazar et al., 2013; Breslau et al., 2004; Copeland et al., 2007). Nearly 13%-33% of them could have suffered multiple traumas (Arata et al., 2005; McLaughlin et al., 2013), an occurrence that was even more severe (62%) among American adolescents in foster care (Salazar et al., 2013). Loss of someone close, physical violence, and traffic accidents were the most commonly reported events in the US (McLaughlin et al., 2013), Denmark (Elklit, 2002), and other European countries (Elklit & Petersen, 2008). The prevalence rates for sexual abuse (1%-15%), physical abuse (5%-50%), emotional abuse (7%-34%), and neglect (34%-59%) were also high among teenagers across countries such as Australia, the US, Canada, Denmark, and the Netherlands (Creighton, 2004; Lampe, 2002).

Turning to adolescents in China, 46%-94% of them reported at least one form of traumatization before the age of eighteen (Wang et al., 2020; Wang & Chung, 2020; Chen & Chung, 2016; Wang et al., 2017; Wang et al., 2021; Yu et al., 2020; Xiao et al., 2021; Chan, 2013) and 14%-58% experienced polyvictimization (Chan, 2013; Wang et al., 2020; Wang & Chung, 2020; Chen & Chung, 2016; Wang et al., 2017; Wang et al., 2021; Yu et al., 2020). The prevalence rates for sexual abuse, physical abuse, emotional abuse, physical neglect, and emotional neglect were 9%-27%, 4%-37%,11%-45%,40%-79%, and 26%-60%, respectively (Wang et al., 2017; Fang et al., 2015; Ji & Finkelhor, 2015; Li et al., 2014; Zhao et al., 2004; Lu et al., 2020; Lin et al., 2011; Yu et al., 2020). These figures estimated among Chinese adolescents were generally comparable to those among overseas youths.

1.1.1.2   Past Trauma, Psychological Distress, and PTSD

Psychological distress includes a number of problematic, confusing and unordinary symptoms, and manifestations of a victim's internal world. Internalizing distress as one aspect of psychological distress implies that victims would like to keep problems to themselves, leading to psychological symptoms including anxiety, depression, withdrawal, dissociation, obsessive-compulsive disorder, trauma and stress-related distress disorders, suicidal ideation, and loneliness (Regier et al., 2013). Externalizing problems are also psychological problems. Different from internalizing distress, externalizing problems are often manifested outward by individuals displaying problematic behaviors such as substance use (e.g., alcohol/drug/cigarette use or dependence), conduct problems (e.g., aggression, delinquency, threatening others, carrying a weapon, deliberately hurting other people, and suicidal attempt), impulsivity, and many other disorders (Krueger et al., 2005).

Trauma could disrupt individuals' psychological functioning and induce and intensify psychological distress. Hence, it is plausible to find traumatized adolescents also reporting heightened feelings of guilt (Szentágotai-Tǎtar & Miu, 2016), impulsivity (Boisseau et al., 2009), psychopathic personality (Farina et al., 2018), and alexithymia (Sayar et al., 2005). A history of trauma exposure was also associated with bipolar disorder (BD) among traumatized adolescents in New Zealand (Rucklidge, 2006).

Additionally, compared with non-traumatized youths, those with past trauma also suffered elevated levels of general psychological distress including depression, anxiety, somatic complaints, dissociation, and other trauma-related symptoms. For instance, at a youth care center in the Netherlands, Meesters et al. (2000) found that adolescents with past trauma reported significantly higher levels of depression than those without such a history. In Canada, Wolfe et al. (2001) observed that high school students with a history of child maltreatment experienced significantly higher levels of anger, depression, anxiety, and dissociation, compared with their counterparts. Later in Sweden, Svedin et al. (2004) found clinical youths who were exposed to past trauma scored significantly higher on the total score of and the four subscales of dissociation than those without trauma exposure; and this result also held true for nonclinical adolescents. Similarly in Turkey, Sayar et al. (2005) revealed a positive association between physical abuse and dissociation, depression, and anxiety within a random sample of adolescent students attending government-run high schools. Subsequently in China, Chung and Chen (2017) examined the relationship between past trauma and psychiatric co-morbidity among vocational school students; adolescents with past trauma reported more psychiatric co-morbid symptoms like depression, anxiety, dissociation, and somatic problems than those without such a stressful experience.

Consistently, researchers in the United States found the same relationship between past trauma and co-morbid symptoms. For example, a history of sexual abuse was associated with traumatic symptoms like anxiety, depression, anger, and dissociation among American adolescents who were receiving psychiatric treatment (Jardin et al., 2017). Childhood trauma was positively associated with mental health issues among a group of juvenile offenders and institutionalized delinquents (Farina et al., 2018). Past trauma was positively associated with depression, anxiety, somatization, obsessive compulsiveness, hostility, psychoticism, paranoia, and interpersonal sensitivity among clinical youths receiving residential treatment for antisocial behaviors in the U. S. (Garland et al., 2013). Similarly, McChesney et al. (2015) found that adolescents in the high-risk groups reported significantly

6

more major depressive episodes, generalized anxiety disorder, and dysthymia symptoms than their counterparts in the low-risk class. In addition, Zeller et al. (2015) found that severely, clinically obese adolescents who were maltreated in childhood suffered more severe internalizing problems of anxiety, depression, withdrawal, and somatic symptoms, compared to their counterparts without maltreatment experience.

The above result was subsequently replicated in a longitudinal study. Gustafsson et al. (2017) focused on a group of healthy pregnant adolescents and found that pregnant adolescents exposed to maternal emotional abuse in childhood reported significantly higher levels of depression at baseline and 37-week follow-up than those without such a trauma exposure.

Another type of distress outcome related to trauma exposure was substance use, such as alcohol abuse or dependence, smoking, marijuana use, drug abuse, and so on. The association between past trauma and substance use has been validated in many empirical studies. For instance, Garland et al. (2013) found adolescents with past trauma were more likely to report substance misuse among a sample receiving residential treatment for antisocial behaviors. Based on two nationally representative adolescent samples in the United States, adolescents exposed to any potential trauma were at higher risks for alcohol and drug abuse (McChesney et al., 2015), and substance use like marijuana, cocaine, prescription drugs, other drugs, and multiple drugs; and the more trauma adolescents were exposed to, the more severe their substance use was (Carliner et al., 2016). Meanwhile, adolescents with alcohol abuse or alcohol dependence reported significantly more childhood abuse (Zeller et al., 2015), physical abuse, sexual abuse, or other adverse life events (Clark et al., 1997), compared with the control group.

In addition, trauma exposure was also found positively related to cigarette use among US adolescents with a history of child maltreatment, emotional abuse, sexual abuse, community violence, or peer victimization (Gooding et al., 2015). Past trauma was also associated with gasoline misuse among a group of American adolescents seeking treatment in the Division of Youth Services (Garland et al., 2011). Most recently, Barry et al. (2019) replicated this within a group of adolescents attending a military-style residential program in the U. S.; being exposed to previous stressful life events was associated with more frequent use of alcohol and marijuana and more other substance use-related problems. Similar results were also documented in a longitudinal study carried out within a group of African-American female juvenile adolescents in the U. S. (Seth et al., 2017); adolescents having experienced community violence reported significantly more marijuana use at baseline and 3-month follow-up.

Suicidality was another possible outcome related to past trauma, either in the form of suicidal ideation or actual suicide behaviors. For example, Kaplow et al. (2014) focused on a clinical adolescent sample seeking treatment for medical or psychiatric problems at an urban medical center in the Midwestern US; adolescents with a history of adverse life events reported stronger suicidal ideation and more suicide behaviors, compared to those without such a stressful history. In exploring the difference in traumatic events between adolescents with suicide ideation and adolescents with suicide behaviors, Plener et al. (2011) found that adolescents with suicide behaviors reported significantly more sexual abuse and multiple trauma exposure than those with suicidal ideation among ninth graders in Germany. However, the researchers did not collect data on the trauma history of adolescents without suicidality, which prevented us from detecting the difference in trauma history between students with and without suicidality. Nevertheless, the above finding was not replicated in Doorley et al. (2017) among a group of psychiatrically hospitalized adolescents in the U. S. ; their adolescents with a history of sexual abuse did not differentiate from those without sexual abuse in the levels of suicide ideation.

There were some other externalizing problems associated with past trauma, such as aggression, unprotected sex, delinquency, and eating disorders. For instance, aggressive and rule-breaking behaviors were found to be associated with child maltreatment among American adolescents (Zeller et al., 2015) and with all types of prior trauma within American adolescent clinical populations (Darnell et al., 2019). Aggression was also related to hurricane exposure even after controlling for proactive aggression (Marsee, 2008). In addition, other misconducts such as carrying weapons secretly and violent or nonviolent delinquent behaviors were also significantly associated with past trauma among high school girls in Canada; threatening behaviors or physical abuse was associated with prior trauma among high school boys (Wolfe et al., 2001), dangerous sex and sexual sensation seeking at baseline, 3-month follow-up, and 6-month follow-up were all associated with a history of community violence among African-American female juvenile adolescents (Seth et al., 2017), and disciplinary infractions were related to prior exposure to stressful life events among US adolescents who attended a military-style residential program (Charles et al., 2019). In addition, abuse-related sleep disturbances at baseline and 37-week follow-up were found positively associated with maternal emotional abuse in childhood among healthy pregnant adolescents in the U. S. (Gustafsson et al., 2017).

Child maltreatment, childhood abuse, and many other adverse life events were associated with various forms of internalizing distress in both Eastern and Western adolescents. This suggests that the negative effects of preceding trauma on adolescents' psychological health were somewhat universal (Chung & Chen, 2017). Adolescents with past trauma were also at higher risk of developing externalizing problems like aggression, delinquency, suicidal attempts, and drug, alcohol, cigarette, or marijuana use, and substance use. This is reasonable given that traumatic events are usually detrimental and out of one's control. Exposure to such uncontrollable events may evoke intense emotional reactions such as anger, and anger may in turn lead to failure to inhibit aggressive reactions (Greenwald, 2002) and trigger oppositional behaviors (Scheeringa & Zeanah, 2008).

Additionally, traumatic events could also affect adolescents' emotion regulation capability, leading to emotional problems (Sayar et al., 2005; Rucklidge, 2006; Garland et al., 2013; Zeller et al., 2015; Darnell et al., 2019). This is not surprising given that traumatic events could impact the neural system that governs the process of emotion regulation (Owens et al., 2012), making traumatized victims (adolescents in this case) more sensitive to emotional conflicts (Marusak et al., 2015). Adolescents might thus become alert to potential dangers, or be passive or submissive to avoid further aggression (Macleod et al, 2002). In this case, an individual might feel helpless, hopeless, and isolated (Browne & Finkelhor, 1986). If the victims had difficulties in regulating and adjusting their emotions, or adopted maladaptive emotional regulation strategies such as responding to the adverse situation implicitly without cognitive engagement (Gross & Munoz, 1995; Gyurak et al., 2011), they would probably suffer greater distress (Chung & Chen, 2017). For example, American adolescents who experienced a prior hurricane reported higher levels of poorly regulated emotions than those without such an experience (Marsee, 2008). Among an American nationally representative sample, adolescents with past trauma reported higher levels of maladaptive coping (Vaughn-Coaxum et al., 2018), and Romanian adolescents with poor emotion regulation skills displayed more depression, anxiety, and guilt symptoms than their counterparts

(Szentágotai-Tătar & Miu, 2016).

Empirical studies also offered support for the mediation of emotion regulation on the relation between traumatic events and psychological distress. For instance, Chung and Chen (2017) found that a history of past trauma was associated with greater emotion-processing difficulties, which in turn was associated with more severe psychiatric co-morbid symptoms among Chinese vocational school students. Likewise, US clinical adolescents with an adverse history were more likely to adopt maladaptive emotion regulation strategies like emotional suppression; and those who adopted emotional suppression in turn reported more suicide thoughts and attempts than their counterparts (Kaplow et al., 2014).

During adolescence, as adolescents undergo biological pubertal changes, their emotion regulation is also experiencing great changes in this special developmental period (Casey, 2015). Maltreatment or abuse from someone close could make the victim feel betrayed (Chung & Chen, 2017). Betrayal from someone close and psychological confusion in adolescence could make adolescents more sensitive to emotional conflicts (Marusak et al., 2015). According to the self-trauma theory (Briere, 2002), trauma would undermine victims' self-capacities in emotion regulation, disrupt the maturation of emotion regulation, heighten the possibility of adopting maladaptive emotion regulation strategies (e.g., suppression, brooding, and worry), and ultimately increase the risks for internalizing (e.g., anxiety and depression) and externalizing problems (e.g., substance use, aggression, and suicide).

Posttraumatic stress disorder (PTSD) is another common sequela in the aftermath of trauma. It can develop among people who have been directly or indirectly exposed to trauma in one of the four forms that have been elucidated earlier (DSM-V, American Psychiatric Association, 2013). This disorder is accompanied by disturbing thoughts and intense feelings about the catastrophizing event even long after the event has been removed. Victims with PTSD might have repeated intrusive memories or dreams about the traumatic event as if they were re-experiencing it; they may feel upset and have strong physical reactions (e.g., sweating and heart pounding) when being reminded of the event, in which case they strive to avoid any of these reminders; they may hold negative beliefs about the self (self-blame) and the world (e.g., The world is dangerous) and be overwhelmed by distressing affects (e.g., fear, sadness, anger, estrangement, and disinterest); also, they may stay hyperalert and act aggressively. These specific PTSD symptoms fall into four symptom clusters: intrusion, avoidance, negative alterations in cognition and mood, and alterations in arousal and reactivity.

Different victims may display different severities of PTSD. According to the DSM-V screening criteria, individuals with no endorsement in any of the four symptom clusters would be given no PTSD; an endorsement in all four symptom clusters would be diagnosed as probable PTSD; and any other cases falling in between the criteria of no PTSD and probable PTSD would be given partial PTSD. The prevalence rate for probable PTSD ranges from 3% to 70% among adolescent survivors of diverse traumas in Western countries (Davis & Siegel, 2000; Galea et al., 2005; Bokszczanin, 2007; Agustini et al., 2011; Deykin & Buka, 1997; Ndetei et al., 2007; Silva et al., 2000; Landolt et al., 2013; Keller et al., 2010; McMillen et al., 2005; Merikangas et al., 2010; Ghazali et al., 2014).

Turning to Chinese adolescents, this rate has been found to vary between 2.5% and 82.6% following a whole range of fearful events (Cao et al., 2015; Ying et al., 2015; Chen & Chung, 2016; Chung & Chen, 2017; Wang et al., 2021; Wang & Chung, 2020; Wang et al., 2020; Quan et al., 2017; Ma et al., 2011; Jin et al., 2019). Taken together, the prevalence rates of probable PTSD among traumatized adolescents in both China and other countries demonstrated large variations, which might result from the differences in PTSD assessment instruments, sample sizes, characteristics of samples under investigation (e.g., clinical or nonclinical, age, and gender), time since trauma, and the nature and severity of trauma (La et al., 1996; Cohen, 1998; Asarnow et al., 1999).

The relationship between trauma exposure and posttraumatic stress disorder has been well-established in the literature. For instance, London et al. (2015) found that a history of child maltreatment was positively associated with PTSD among adolescents in the United States. Similarly, McChesney et al. (2015) adopted latent class analysis among a large nationally representative adolescent sample in the U. S., grouped adolescents into four different classes based on their patterns of traumatic experiences, and revealed that except for the low-risk group (not likely to experience any trauma), all other three classes (the sexual assault risk group, the non-sexual risk group, and the high-risk group) reported significantly higher levels of PTSD. Most recently, also in America, Darnell et al. (2019) focused on a group of clinical adolescents and found that past trauma was positively associated with posttraumatic stress disorder regardless of trauma type. American clinical adolescents who were sexually abused (Jardin et al., 2017) and American high school students who had experienced a hurricane (Marsee, 2008) also reported elevated PTSD distress.

Apart from the studies in the U. S., one cross-sectional investigation conducted in Canada also revealed that adolescents with a history of child maltreatment, regardless of gender, had much higher risks of developing posttraumatic stress symptoms compared with their counterparts who did not experience any trauma (Wolfe et al., 2001). The same result was replicated in a longitudinal study by Seth et al.(2017). They followed up a group of African-American female adolescents exposed to prior community violence for six months, measured posttraumatic stress disorder at three time points, and found that community violence was marginally associated with PTSD at baseline but significantly predicted PTSD at both 3-month follow-up and 6-month follow-up. This positive relationship between PTSD and past trauma was quite consistent in the literature, although different studies used different measures and different diagnostic criteria to evaluate PTSD.

1.1.2　Past Trauma and Positive Psychological Changes

1.1.2.1　Positive Psychological Changes

It has long been documented that trauma reactions are not limited to the pattern of psychopathology. Rather, something positive could also emerge from fearful experiences (Waysman et al., 2001; Linley & Joseph, 2004). This was not only reflected by the old teachings of religions in Eastern and Western cultures (e.g., Buddhism, Hinduism, Islam, and Christianity) that propounded human suffering possesses transformative power and could be the origin of significant good (e. g., humanity, wisdom, truth, and spirituality) (Tedeschi et al., 1995) but also by evidence from subsequent trauma research (Ai & Park, 2005). Previously, there was no consistent term for this type of phenomenon, which was initially called "positive illusions" (Taylor & Brown, 1988). Later on, when it was recognized by more and more psychiatrists and researchers, it gradually became known as "positive psychological changes" (Yalom & Lieberman, 1991), "perceived benefits" or "construing benefits" (Calhoun & Tedeschi, 1991; McMillen et al., 1995; Tennen et al., 1992), "thriving" (O'Leary & Ickovics, 1995), "stress-related growth" (Park et al., 1996), adversarial growth (Linley & Joseph, 2004), flourishing (Ryff & Singer, 1998), and discovery of meaning (Bower et al., 1998). Subsequently, it was proposed that the term "posttraumatic growth" (PTG) might best capture this positive pattern of traumatic reactions, as posttraumatic growth reflects self-transcending and better psychological functioning exceeding previous levels of adaptation (Tedeschi et al., 1998).

1.1.2.2   Posttraumatic Growth among Adolescents

It is the struggle in coping with trauma and its negative effects that really matters for PTG development, rather than the traumatic event itself (Tedeschi & Calhoun, 1995). Posttraumatic growth is defined in terms of the positive changes that victims can experience following a trauma (Tedeschi & Calhoun, 1995). Whilst trauma can disrupt cognitive processes, core beliefs, and assumptive worldviews and disorganize the self-structure, which gives rise to a new traumatized self-structure, it can also lead victims to reconstruct their lives, to rebuild the world assumptions shattered by the trauma (Tedeschi & Calhoun, 1996; Boals & Schuettler, 2011; Barton et al., 2013), and to display "fully functioning" characteristics including a desire for social organizations, trusting relationships, and compassion for others (Joseph, 2012). Improvement in personal strengths, appreciation for life, new possibilities, and spiritual change could also emerge among victims (Tedeschi & Calhoun, 1996). Greater personal strengths include greater self-reliance and self-capacities in handling life issues; increased appreciation of life implies re-organized life priorities and enhanced valuing of daily life; new possibilities connote new interests, life paths and opportunities, as well as necessary changes as a result of the fearful experience; and spiritual changes signify deeper religious faith and a stronger sense of harmony with the universe (Tedeschi & Calhoun, 1996).

However, in addition to treating PTG traditionally as an outcome of the struggle with trauma, the formulation of action-focused growth (Hobfoll et al., 2007) and the Janus-face model of PTG (Maercker & Zoellner, 2004) suggest PTG could also be a kind of coping strategy for dealing with trauma. PTG has two components: the authentic self-transcending growth and the illusory self-deceptive growth (Maercker & Zoellner, 2004). The former (authentic growth) promotes post-trauma adaptation and constructive psychological functioning, and the latter (illusory growth) impedes post-event adjustment and intensifies psychological distress in the long run.

The last few years have seen much effort in distinguishing PTG from resilience. Resilience previously refers to a dynamic developmental process reflecting evidence of positive adaptation despite significant life adversity (Masten, 2014). However, this definition shares many similarities with posttraumatic growth. With the development of PTG research stepping into a distinct area, the other definition of resilience is more broadly recognized and accepted, i.e., the ability to recover from or adjust easily to adversity or misfortune (Tedeschi & Kilmer, 2005). To be specific, resilience is the ability to overcome adversity and return back to normal functioning in the short run (Scales et al., 2000).

PTG and resilience are distinct from each other in the following three aspects. Firstly, PTG is about self-transcending and moving beyond pre-trauma levels of functioning across dimensions including self-perceptions, relationship with others, and life philosophy, but resilience is about being unaffected by trauma and bouncing back to the previous state of functioning (Meyerson et al., 2011; Clay et al., 2009). Secondly, whilst PTG may often coexist with psychological distress like posttraumatic stress disorder (PTSD) and other symptomatology, resilience reflects adaptation, reduction, or even absence of psychopathological symptoms when confronted with traumatic life events (Meyerson et al., 2011; Clay et al., 2009; Scales et al., 2000). Finally, individuals who are resilient are not necessarily more likely to experience PTG. As PTG requires some degree of psychological distress, traumatization, and cognitive struggle (Calhoun & Tedeschi, 2006), those resilient but not traumatized (or distressed) individuals may be less likely to grow (Clay et al., 2009).

Previous research mainly adopted the following five types of instruments to measure posttraumatic growth among adolescents and children. The strengths and weaknesses of each instrument were discussed.

1) The Posttraumatic Growth Inventory (PTGI; Tedeschi & Calhoun, 1996) was initially developed for traumatized adults, with 21 items measuring positive outcomes across five domains: "new possibilities", "relating to others", "personal strength", "spiritual change", and "appreciation of life". A further confirmatory factor analysis (CFA) supported this five-factor model (Taku et al., 2008). Good reliability, validity, and internal consistency were also achieved (Tedeschi & Calhoun, 1996). This scale proved to be useful in measuring adults' successful struggle with trauma and its aftermath (Tedeschi & Calhoun, 1996). Although it is later broadly used in many empirical studies among children and adolescents, several weaknesses must be mentioned. First, the wording might be difficult for young people (adolescents in this case) to fully understand the items (e. g., "I established a new path for my life.") (Ickovics et al., 2006). Second, all items are positively worded (e.g., "I discovered that I'm stronger than I thought I was.") (Milam et al., 2004; Boals & Schuler, 2018). Third, its 6-point Likert response scale mainly allows for positive reports ("0 = did not experience this change"; "1 = experienced this change to a very small degree"; "2 = experienced this change to a small degree"; "3 = experienced this change to a moderate degree"; "4 = experienced this change to a great degree"; "5 = experienced this change to a very great degree") (Milam et al., 2004; Boals & Schuler, 2018).

2) The modified PTGI (Milam et al., 2004) was adapted from the PTGI, with 16 items assessing posttraumatic growth among traumatized adolescents from the same five dimensions as PTGI. Items were modified and reworded to be easily understood by adolescents. The 6-point Likert response scale was also modified to allow for options of positive/no/negative change. Good internal consistency reliability was reported. Whilst encouraging, further validation tests and confirmatory factor analyses are unavailable and need to be examined in future studies (Clay et al., 2009).

3) The modified PTGI (Ickovics et al., 2006) was also adapted from the PTGI for use among adolescents, with 19 items covering four domains of the PTGI: "new possibilities", "relating to others", "personal strength", and "appreciation of life". The two items for "spiritual change" were deleted as they were thought not applicable to adolescents. To enhance comprehension among adolescents, items were simplified (e.g., "Appreciating each day" became "You realized that each day is important"), and the scoring system was shortened to a 3-point (6-point in original) Likert scale (0 = no change, 1 = a little change, 2 = a lot of change). Although the modified scale possessed good internal consistency reliability, and the 4-factor model was reached by confirmatory factor analysis, its validity is still of greater concern. Besides, the two items for "spiritual change" domain may not necessarily need to be dropped as adolescents in other cultures might have a greater sense of religious issues.

4) The Posttraumatic Growth Inventory for Children (PTGI-C; Cryder et al., 2006) was also adapted from the PTGI, with 21 items covering the same five domains as the original scale. Words and content were modified. Good internal consistency reliability was supported by preliminary data, but the validity of the scale was not reported.

5) The Revised Posttraumatic Growth Inventory for Children (PTGI-C-

R；Kilmer et al., 2009) was adapted from PTGI-C，with 10 items and 2 open-ended questions covering the same five aspects of PTGI. To facilitate comprehension and application among children and adolescents，the wording and language were modified and simplified，an introduction with additional explanation and two open-ended questions were incorporated，certain items were dropped，and the scoring system was also shortened to a 4-point scale (0 ＝ no change；1 ＝ a little change；2 ＝ some change；3＝a lot of change). This scale showed good reliability and construct validity.

Traumatic events shatter individuals' existing world assumptions, challenge their pre-schema and core beliefs about themselves，others，and the world，force them to alter previous worldviews and core beliefs, and reconstruct post-event schema to promote the development of PTG (Tedeschi ＆ Calhoun, 2004). In light of the comprehensive model of posttraumatic growth (Calhoun ＆ Tedeschi，2006) and the model of assumptive worlds (Janoff-Bulman，1989)，the key issue for achieving PTG lies in whether the victims cognitively ruminate about trauma and its clues. Intrusive rumination functions to increase psychological distress which triggers victims to deliberately ruminate about trauma. Deliberate rumination facilitates the task-relevant problem-solving processes, constructively analyzes trauma information，reconciles trauma with their representation world，integrates trauma into their self-structure，and extracts meaning from this fearful experience.

However，these posttraumatic cognitive processes could be affected by prior-trauma factors (e.g., gender, ethnicity, personality, and resilience), factors at the time of trauma (e.g., trauma type and trauma exposure severity)，and post-trauma factors (e.g., social support，positive affect，age, socioeconomic status，and time since trauma).

Prior-trauma factors

Gender

Although one study reported a higher level of posttraumatic growth among their male participants (Du et al., 2018), one revealed higher levels of PTG among females (Wu et al., 2018), and another study failed to find any significant gender difference in posttraumatic growth among traumatized adolescents (An et al., 2018). Notwithstanding this, a longitudinal study reported mixed results: females reported significantly more PTG than males at T1, but this gender difference became nonsignificant at T4 (Ying et al., 2014).

Some of the above studies failed to find any gender difference in posttraumatic growth, which is consistent with the findings from a systematic review (Meyerson et al., 2011). PTG requires traumatization and cognitive rumination (Tedeschi & Calhoun, 1995). Although females around puberty were more likely to be exposed to negative interpersonal events and ruminate about them (Hankin & Abramson, 2001), it took time for gender differences in PTG to become more pronounced, around the age of 35, in general (Vishnevsky et al., 2010). This implies that the nonsignificant relation between gender and PTG might be because gender differences have not emerged yet. Although one study identified a higher level of PTG among males, it may have some relation with males' greater sense of responsibility and more chances for growth (Du et al., 2018). The other study reported a higher level of PTG among females; this could be because females are more likely to make efforts in interpersonal interactions which then enables them to experience greater growth in relationships with others (Wu et al., 2018; Belle, 1991). For another, females' higher sensitivity to themselves, others, and the world might have facilitated deliberate rumination about trauma and schema alteration which is required for growth (Cryder et al., 2006).

20

Ethnicity

Two studies examined the relationship between ethnicity and posttraumatic growth eight years following the 2008 Wenchuan earthquake (Du et al., 2018; Wu et al., 2018). Both studies revealed significant differences in PTG between the Han and non-Han ethnic groups in the severely affected area; the Han ethnic group reported significantly lower levels of posttraumatic growth than the non-Han ethnic groups. This might have some relation with the special cultural and spiritual life of the non-Han ethnic minorities (Proffitt et al., 2007; Maguen et al., 2006; Laufer & Solomon, 2006). These minority adolescents were mainly from the Qiang and Zang ethnic groups. The former (Qiang) emphasizes toughness and tolerance which might help adolescents fight against trauma and grow from it. The latter (Zang) believes in Buddhism and religious individuals are more likely to experience growth than nonreligious one (Laufer & Solomon, 2006).

However, the above ethnic difference in PTG did not emerge among participants in the generally affected area (Du et al., 2018). This might be owing to the low variance of samples' ethnicities in the generally affected area. Nearly all participants (98.6%) were Han people in this area, compared with 52.7% of Han people in the severely affected area (Du et al., 2018).

Personality

Personality, as a relatively stable psychological resource, was assumed to play an important role in the development of posttraumatic growth (Zerach, 2015). However, only one study has investigated the relationship between personality dimensions and PTG among traumatized adolescents (An et al., 2017). Based on the big-five model of personality (Costa & McCrae, 1992), the researchers found posttraumatic growth was directly positively associated with extraversion, openness, agreeableness, and conscientiousness, but not related to neuroticism (An et al., 2017). In addition, most dimensions of personality also predicted PTG via positive cognition coping (An et al., 2017).

Positive cognition coping was a significant predictor for PTG and was highly associated with most PTG domains (Bellizzi & Blank, 2006). Stable human traits like personality might use positive cognition coping to fight against trauma, thereby producing positive changes (An et al., 2017). For instance, the extravert and agreeable adolescents may be more inclined to accept and adopt positive coping strategies, e.g., positive cognition coping, which stimulates individuals to deliberately ruminate about trauma and its aftermath and find meaning from trauma.

Resilience

Evidence of resilience to be a protective factor for posttraumatic growth was documented in the literature. Two studies reported a positive relationship between resilience and posttraumatic growth concurrently (Yuan et al., 2018; Levine et al., 2009), although Levine et al. (2009) operationalized resilience with a lack of PTSD. This positive relationship was subsequently replicated in a longitudinal study (Zhou et al., 2015). Specifically, T1 resilience significantly predicted T2 PTG even after controlling for age and T1 PTG, but T2 resilience did not predict T3 PTG (Zhou et al., 2015). Additionally, some studies focused on adolescents' trait resilience and found trait resilience was also positively associated with PTG among Chinese adolescents 12 months following the Wenchuan earthquake (Ying et al., 2016) and among Japanese adolescents exposed to negative life events after controlling for time since the negative event (Nishikawa et al., 2018).

Thus, resilience might facilitate posttraumatic growth among traumatized adolescents. This is reasonable given that resilient individuals are more flexible in emotion regulation (Waugh et al., 2008). They reconcile self-anticipation with situational needs and regulate affective responses accordingly. Resilient individuals were also less inclined to generalize negative impacts of one situation to others, thus reducing resource consumption (Zhou et al., 2015). More resources (psychological, social, and physical) were then available for fighting against trauma to facilitate growth (Zhou et al., 2015; Hobfoll, 1989). In addition, this flexibility in regulating negative emotions also enables individuals to shift attention from the negative context of trauma to constructive task-relevant stimuli, i.e., cognitive reappraisal and deliberate rumination, thus creating meaning from trauma and its aftermath (Koster et al., 2011).

Factors at the time of trauma

Type of trauma

One prospective study investigated the impact of different trauma types on posttraumatic growth (Vloet et al., 2014). Compared with victims of non-sexual abuse, survivors of sexual abuse reported significantly higher levels of PTG at follow-up. This finding contradicted the other research (Ickovics et al., 2006) in that survivors of natural disasters were more likely to experience PTG than victims of "human-made" trauma, i.e., sexual abuse and interpersonal violence, as "human-made" trauma, perceived as controllable and preventable, is much more psychologically devastating than natural disasters. The inconsistency between the above two studies might be due to the effect of the intervention treatment (Hagenaars & van Minnen, 2010). In fact, almost all sexually abused victims in Vloet et al. (2014) had received a certain period of professional psychotherapy before data collection took place.

Exposure severity

The relation between trauma exposure severity and posttraumatic growth was not without controversy. Among the studies that measured trauma exposure severity with the Trauma Severity Questionnaire (Wu et al., 2013), most reported a positive concurrent relation between these two variables (Zhou et al., 2018; Zhou et al., 2017; Zhou et al., 2016), and one found a nonsignificant relation (Tian et al., 2018).

Among the two studies that assessed trauma exposure severity differently, one reported that earthquake survivors in the severely affected area obtained significantly higher scores on the total score and the subscales of PTGI than victims in the generally affected area (Du et al., 2018). This suggests a positive relation between trauma severity and posttraumatic growth. However, when examining the relationship between these two constructs separately in the severely affected and generally affected areas, quite a different story emerged. Specifically, neither being buried oneself nor the death of a family member was significantly associated with PTG in each of the two areas (Du et al., 2018). It might be the homogeneous sample (predominantly adolescents neither being buried themselves nor having a family member dead) in both areas that constricted variances and diminished the relation among variables. However, the house collapse was associated with PTG for the severely affected area only (Du et al., 2018). This might be due to the high variance (16.1%) of house collapse in the severely affected area (that of the generally affected area: 0.6%).

The other was a prospective study, measuring trauma exposure severity with the Earthquake Exposure Questionnaire (Chen et al., 2002) at T1 and PTG at T1 and T2 (Ying et al., 2014). The researchers found that indirect exposure was significantly positively correlated with T1 and T2 PTG, and worry about others was positively associated with T1 PTG only. Neither direct exposure nor house damage was associated with PTG at any time point.

In addition to trauma exposure severity, one study examined the relationship between the palpitation and anxiety victims felt during trauma and their scores on the PTGI (Du et al., 2018). Evidence showed that survivors experiencing a higher level of palpitation and anxiety when the earthquake took place reported significantly higher levels of PTG eight years later. The other investigation measured the stress Japanese adolescents experienced at the time of the negative life event (NLE) and examined the relationship between this stress and posttraumatic growth separately within boys and girls (Nishikawa et al., 2018). The stress at the time of trauma was positively associated with PTG across gender.

To sum up, most studies investigating the relationship between trauma exposure severity and posttraumatic growth reported a positive relation between these two constructs. This echoed a previous review among children and adolescents (Meyerson et al., 2011). Evidence of a positive relation between PTG and psychological distress at the time of trauma, including stress (Nishikawa et al., 2018), palpitation, and anxiety (Du et al., 2018), also emerged. These findings supported the assumption that some degree of psychological distress from trauma was a prerequisite for posttraumatic growth (Tedeschi & Calhoun, 2004).

Post-trauma factors

Rumination and Core beliefs

Rumination might also affect the development of posttraumatic growth. Findings regarding the relationship between deliberate rumination (i.e., purposeful problem-solving, one type of rumination) and PTG were quite consistent across studies. Deliberate rumination was positively associated with posttraumatic growth even after controlling for social support (Zhou et al., 2014). Besides, the cross-lagged panel model from a longitudinal study revealed that deliberate rumination and PTG predicted each other reciprocally over time (T1 and T2 deliberate rumination significantly predicted T2 and T3 PTG, respectively, and vice versa), even after controlling for T1, T2, & T3 PTSD, prior and subsequent deliberate rumination, and earlier and later PTG (Wu et al., 2015). By contrast, intrusive rumination (e.g., unintentional brooding) was documented as negatively associated with posttraumatic growth (Xu et al., 2019; Zhou et al., 2014); and the impact of intrusive rumination on posttraumatic growth was mediated by deliberate rumination (Zhou et al., 2014).

The above relationship between rumination and posttraumatic growth supported the previous view that rumination affects PTG through its content (constructive and unconstructive components) rather than its amount (Cryder et al., 2006; Watkins, 2008). Indeed, deliberate rumination (the constructive and productive component) was a significant protective factor for PTG in all three studies that examined these two constructs (Xu et al., 2019; Zhou et al., 2014; Wu et al., 2015). Whilst intrusive rumination (the negative and unconstructive component) was not correlated with PTG in Pearson correlation (Xu et al., 2019; Zhou et al., 2014), intrusive rumination significantly predicted PTG directly and indirectly via deliberate rumination in further structural equation modeling after controlling for core beliefs (Zhou et al., 2014).

The more victims' core beliefs were challenged, the higher levels of PTG they might experience. In light of the assumptive world model (Janoff-Bulman, 1989) and the comprehensive model of PTG (Calhoun & Tedeschi, 2006), trauma challenges adolescents' core beliefs about themselves, others, and the world. This disparity between prior-and-post trauma core beliefs causes cognitive conflict, to make sense of which adolescents have to ruminate about trauma clues. Deliberate rumination facilitates adolescents to focus on the positive task-relevant stimuli and adopt problem-solving strategies, promotes their understanding of the self, others, and the world, and creates meaning from trauma and its aftermath to foster PTG.

By contrast, intrusive rumination (a passive cognitive activity) forces negative thoughts about the self and trauma into adolescents' cognitive world, which takes up working memory and immerses adolescents in the negative context of trauma, causing huge psychological distress and hindering problem-solving and the development of PTG. However, some researchers argued that the psychological pressure accruing from intrusive rumination might in turn stimulate deliberate rumination about trauma and its pathogenic effects to relieve pressure (Joseph & Linley, 2004; Butler et al., 2005). Thus, intrusive rumination could be a double-edged sword for PTG among adolescents (Zhou et al., 2014).

Other coping strategies

Coping appeared to have a significant effect on adolescents' posttraumatic growth based on the evidence of two studies that examined the relationship between different coping strategies and PTG. For instance, positive coping strategies like positive cognition coping (An et al., 2017) and active coping (Du et al., 2018) were positively associated with PTG. This echoed prior literature in that active coping strategies were significant predictors of PTG (Meyerson et al., 2011). These findings supported the PTG theory implying that deliberate rumination lays the foundation for positive reappraisal and reinterpretation of trauma and its aftermath to reconfigure the post-trauma schema regarding oneself, others, and the world for PTG development (Tedeschi & Calhoun, 1995; Joseph & Linley, 2004). Passive coping was negatively related to the development of posttraumatic growth (Du et al., 2018), suggesting maladaptive coping has deleterious effects on growth.

With respect to emotion regulation, utilizing cognitive reappraisal dealing with traumatic challenges predicted greater PTG among Chinese adolescents 6 months following the Ya'an earthquake (Zhou et al., 2017;

Zhou et al., 2016) and 8.5 years following the Wenchuan earthquake (Tian et al., 2018), even after controlling for trauma exposure severity, demographic variables (e.g. , age, gender), social support, etc. However, using expressive suppression did not have any effect on the development of growth (Tian et al., 2018; Zhou et al., 2017; Zhou et al., 2016). According to the process model of emotion (Gross, 1998), adolescents adopting a cognitive reappraisal strategy (antecedent-focused) would reappraise and reinterpret trauma and its impact by altering their pre-trauma cognitions to rebuild the meaning of the world, thereby fostering post-trauma adaptation and growth. On the contrary, individuals using an expressive suppression strategy (response-focused) tend to suppress their emotions, which does not involve any cognitive processing like reappraisal and may hamper the development of PTG.

Also, one study examined the relationship between T1 control beliefs and T1 & T2 PTG (Ying et al., 2014). Regression equations showed that T1 primary control beliefs (manipulating the environment to fit for oneself) were only able to predict T1 PTG but not T2 PTG; T1 secondary control beliefs (adjusting oneself to accommodate the environment) positively predicted both T1 and T2 PTG. Both primary and secondary control beliefs were significant predictors of PTG among Chinese adolescents, suggesting the adaptive functions of control beliefs in the wake of trauma (Heckhausen et al., 2010). Notably, primary control (very similar to problem-solving) is adaptive only when goals or the environment is attainable or manipulatable. Otherwise, adolescents, especially in a collectivist culture like China, would resort to secondary control beliefs to adjust cognitions, values, and attributions, aiming to accommodate to the environment and extract meaning from the traumatic event (Heckhausen et al., 2010; Ying et al., 2014). However, research in this field is very limited. Future studies should examine the role control beliefs play in the development of posttraumatic growth.

The role trait mindfulness plays in the development of PTG was also explored in the literature. Trait mindfulness only positively predicted new possibilities and appreciation of life, but not the PTGI total score or other domains of PTG among adolescents exposed to a tornado in China in a cross-sectional study (Xu et al., 2018). This result was replicated in a longitudinal investigation among participants exposed to the same tornado. T1 mindfulness did not predict T1 or T2 PTGI total score (An et al., 2018).

These findings contradicted previous research among college students and adults in that mindfulness was positively associated with PTG (Hanley et al., 2017; Hanley et al., 2015). Mindfulness, a multidimensional construct, refers to paying attention to the present moment on purpose and not judgmentally (Kabat-Zinn, 1994). In light of the mindfulness-to-meaning theory (Garland et al., 2015), mindfulness helps individuals realize that trauma offers the chance for growth, which could facilitate the meaning-making process necessary for the development of PTG. Similarly, mindfulness aids in buffering against deleterious posttraumatic outcomes and extracting meaning from trauma (Hanley et al., 2015). The disparity between Hanley's investigation and the above two studies, i.e., Xu et al. (2018) and An et al. (2018), might be due to the differences in samples under investigation and the measurement instruments for mindfulness. Hanley's studies used a multidimensional scale for mindfulness, while Xu et al. (2018) and An et al. (2018) adopted a unidimensional questionnaire which may not fully capture the construct of "mindfulness". Compared with samples of college students and adults in Hanley's studies, the adolescent samples in Xu et al. (2018) and An et al. (2018) may not be able to apply mindfulness as a coping strategy due to their underdeveloped cognitive function. Therefore, the inadequate capture or under-application of mindfulness might explain why mindfulness was not related to PTG in the other two studies.

Social support

Some studies investigated the relationship between social support and posttraumatic growth. Generally, evidence of a positive relation was revealed. The total score and all five subscales (emotional support, instrumental support, companionship, affirmative evaluation, and intimacy) of social support were positively correlated with the PTGI total score and its three subscales (perceived changes in self, a changed sense of relationships with others, and philosophy of life changes) (Xu et al., 2019). Social support also positively predicted posttraumatic growth (Xu et al., 2019; Zhou et al., 2018; Yuan et al., 2018; Zhou et al., 2017; Zhou et al., 2016; Zhou et al., 2014; Du et al., 2018), even after controlling for trauma exposure, demographic variables, rumination, emotion regulation, attachment, coping, core beliefs, resilience, hope, and self-efficacy. In light of Lepore and Greenberg's theory (2002), social support builds a supportive environment for traumatized adolescents with sufficient physical, psychological, and social resources, to help shift attention from the negative aftermath of trauma to the positive problem-solving stimuli. The latter could facilitate constructive rumination about trauma and associated meaning-making, promoting the development of posttraumatic growth.

Preliminary evidence also emerged regarding the function of parental attachment in promoting PTG following traumatic events among traumatized adolescents. Adolescents with a higher degree of secure attachment reported significantly higher levels of posttraumatic growth 12 months after the Yancheng tornado (Yuan et al., 2018) and 8.5 years after the Wenchuan earthquake (Tian et al., 2018) in China. Thus, attachment to significant others might be a protective mechanism for PTG (Mikulincer & Shaver,

2007). Specifically, secure parental attachment constructs the feelings of being loved, respected, understood, and supported by parents, which help stabilize one's emotions and increase the likelihood of constructive processing about trauma and its outcomes (Fredrickson, 2001), thus facilitating growth.

Other positive psychological constructs

One study examined the effects hope and self-esteem had on posttraumatic growth among adolescents and found that hope directly predicted PTG and self-esteem indirectly predicted PTG via hope (Zhou et al., 2018). Consistent with the hope theory (Snyder, 2002), self-esteem increases hope through motivating adolescents to attain goals by using effective and adaptive coping strategies (Setliff & Marmurek, 2002). Higher levels of hope might then stimulate positive thinking about trauma, oneself, others, and the world (Benzein & Berg, 2005), and facilitate reconfiguration of the post-trauma schema to foster PTG (Calhoun & Tedeschi, 2006).

One study explored the role of self-efficacy on PTG among adolescents and suggested that self-efficacy was another positive predictor for PTG (An et al., 2018). In light of the self-regulation shift theory (Benight et al., 2017), enhanced self-efficacy strengthens individuals' ability in regulating posttraumatic needs and increases the likelihood of constructing positive meaning of the posttraumatic world to promote personal growth (King et al., 2000).

The association between life satisfaction and posttraumatic growth was also explored. These two constructs were positively correlated (Wu et al., 2018). This is reasonable because PTG reflects positive changes in personal strengths, new possibilities, relationships with others, spiritual change, and appreciation of life (Tedeschi & Calhoun, 1996), which could improve individuals' subjective happiness and meaning in life (Triplett et al., 2012), leading to increased satisfaction in life. However, the underlying mechanism between PTG and life satisfaction still needs further investigation, as the current finding was only based on correlation analysis (Wu et al., 2018).

One study examined the function of gratitude on the development of PTG and reported gratitude as a protective factor for posttraumatic growth among adolescents (Zhou and Wu, 2016). According to the broaden-and-build theory of positive emotions (Fredrickson, 2001), gratitude as a positive emotion could broaden adolescents' attention, enabling individuals to pay attention to other possibilities of trauma (e.g., positive changes) rather than being fixed on the negative context of trauma (Fredrickson & Branigan, 2005). Gratitude could also broaden individuals' cognition; the broadening of cognition facilitates cognitive processes including active rumination and integration of trauma into one's existing schema, to make PTG possible (Martin & Clore, 2001). Also, gratitude could trigger constructive behaviors and actions, e.g., adopting more effective and adaptive coping strategies to promote PTG (Fredrickson & Cohn, 2008). In addition, gratitude could also improve the relationship with others (Algoe, 2005), and build and accumulate the psychological and social resources necessary for the development of posttraumatic growth during one's struggle with trauma (Fredrickson, 2001).

Negative psychological constructs

Psychological distress could affect the development of posttraumatic growth. Specifically, posttraumatic fear (Zhou et al., 2018) and depression (Xu et al., 2018) positively predicted PTG. Grief reactions and PTG were also positively correlated (Hirooka et al., 2017). These findings support PTG theory in that some degree of distress is a prerequisite for PTG (Tedeschi & Calhoun, 2004). Limited research tested PTG as a predictor and found PTG predicted the reduction in depression (Nishikawa et al.,

2018；Wu et al., 2018), current stress from previous negative life events (Nishikawa et al., 2018), and academic burnout at T1 (Ying et al., 2016). In light of the formulation of action-focused growth (Hobfoll, 2007) and the Janus-face model of PTG (Maercker & Zoellner, 2004), PTG hereby might represent the constructive self-transcending growth and act as an adaptive way of coping in buffering against psychological distress.

Time since event

Surprisingly, time since event did not significantly impact the development of posttraumatic growth among a group of clinical adolescents (Vloet et al., 2014). This could be due to that almost all participants in Vloet's study received a period of psychotherapy before the assessment was administered; the effects of treatment might have surpassed and covered that of time since event on PTG.

Other demographic variables

The relationship between age or age-related variables (e.g., grade) and posttraumatic growth was inconsistent within traumatized adolescents. Overall, adolescents' experience of PTG was independent of their age (i.e., the age at the time of data collection) (Zhou et al., 2018; Xu et al., 2018; An et al., 2018; Wu et al., 2018; Ying et al., 2014). Two studies found a positive relation between PTG and age (i.e., the age at the time the negative life event happened) (Nishikawa et al., 2018; Ying et al., 2016). Hence, it was the age at the time of the negative event rather than the time of data collection that could significantly predict subsequent posttraumatic growth. Furthermore, taking into consideration that the level of PTG might change as time since trauma passes, researchers proposed that future studies examining the impact of age on the development of PTG should focus on adolescents' age when the traumatic event happened rather than the age when the measurement was administered (Meyerson et al., 2011).

Additionally, the impact of SES and current housing on posttraumatic growth was also explored within a sample of adolescent earthquake survivors in previous studies (Du et al., 2018). Neither a significant difference in PTG was found among adolescents from various SES backgrounds, nor did evidence of a relation between current housing and PTG emerge (Du et al., 2018). These findings echoed the results of a previous review among children and adolescents (Meyerson et al., 2011). It might be the homogeneous sample used (predominantly adolescents from middle-to-high SES families and living in their original houses) that limited the variances in variables and diminished the ability to detect relations among constructs (Meyerson et al., 2011).

1. 1. 2. 3   Past Trauma, PTSD, and Posttraumatic Growth

The relationship between PTSD and posttraumatic growth among adolescents is not without controversy. Whilst PTSD symptoms have been positively associated with posttraumatic growth among adolescents exposed to a whole range of traumas (Alisic et al., 2008; Barakat et al., 2006; Hafstad et al., 2010, 2011; Kilmer & Gil-Rivas, 2010; Kilmer et al., 2009; Laufer & Solomon, 2006; Laufer et al., 2009; Levine et al., 2008; Du et al., 2018; Tian et al., 2016; Yu et al., 2010; Zhou et al., 2015), this relationship has not been established among adolescents in the Gaza Strip (Murad & Thabet, 2017), Jewish Israeli youth (Laufer et al., 2009), or Chinese adolescents exposed to the Ya'an earthquake, (Zhou et al., 2016), the Wenchuan earthquake (Zhou et al., 2018), and the Yancheng tornado (Yuan et al., 2018). Even when the association between PTSD and posttraumatic growth was established, a longitudinal study revealed that the relationship was negative in nature (Chen et al., 2015). Other researchers also found evidence of a significant inverted-U curvilinear relation between PTSD symptoms and posttraumatic growth among Israeli youth following terror exposure (Levine et al., 2008).

These inconsistencies might have confirmed previous PTG theories suggesting that different levels of distress could relate to the development of posttraumatic growth in different ways (Butler et al., 2005; Nelson, 2011; Tedeschi & Calhoun, 2004). This makes sense given that low levels of distress were not upsetting enough to challenge one's world assumptions and core beliefs, which therefore may not trigger growth. Whereas high levels of distress were so overwhelming that they exceeded victims' tolerance capacities. Therefore, victims might develop emotional numbness or cognitive and behavioral avoidance to temporarily escape trauma cues and concomitant negative affects, rather than process these cues. This could undermine meaning-making and posttraumatic growth. However, in the context of moderate levels of distress, the negative emotional arousals were relatively much more easily modulated and tolerated. This tolerance of distress paved the way for and set in motion the subsequent cognitive processing of trauma materials, which in turn could contribute to the emergence of PTG. Nevertheless, these inconsistent findings between PTSD and posttraumatic growth among adolescents warrant further investigation.

Treatment of PTSD to facilitate PTG

One cross-sectional study investigated the role of receiving psychological aid in promoting posttraumatic growth and found that adolescents who had received psychological treatment after being exposed to the Wenchuan earthquake obtained significantly higher scores on the PTGI (Du et al., 2018). A similar finding was replicated in a longitudinal study, where receiving treatment (a trauma-focused cognitive-behavioral therapy) for a period positively predicted T2 posttraumatic growth among a clinical adolescent sample with past trauma (Vloet et al., 2014). However, there was a lack of pretest of PTG in both studies, and detailed information regarding the content, the procedure, as well as the number of treatment sessions was not reported in the two studies.

Another study designed and implemented a 3-week school-based psychoeducational intervention program (learning PTG knowledge, see Taku et al. (2017) for details) among two samples of nonclinical Japanese adolescents. For the first sample (exclusively females), whilst adolescents having received the intervention (learning PTG knowledge) reported significantly higher levels of PTG than those who had not, it remained unclear how PTG knowledge would benefit perceptions of PTG (Taku et al., 2017). To address some of the limitations in the first study, the second study including both male and female participants partly confirmed the effect of the intervention. Specifically, Experimental Group 1 (learning about PTG) reported the highest level of PTG knowledge followed by Experimental Group 2 (learning about PTSD) and the control group (learning about branches, careers, and history of psychology). However, except for the significantly low level of PTG reported by Experimental Group 2, no significant difference in PTG was observed between Experimental Group 1 and the control group (Taku et al., 2017).

The other dissertation implemented and tested a three-session expressive writing intervention among a group of adolescents whose parents were diagnosed with cancer. Adolescents were randomly and evenly assigned to the experimental group (writing about thoughts and feelings about parents' cancer) and the control group (writing about what they did the previous day) (see Laub Huizenga (2011) and Pennebaker (1993) for more details). Pretest, post-test, and follow-up test were administered. The experimental group experienced significantly higher levels of PTG than the control group (Laub Huizenga, 2011).

In summary, past research has witnessed high prevalence rates of traumatic events and concomitant PTSD symptoms among adolescents across the world, which underscores the necessity for more investigation into the impact of trauma on youths' psychological functioning. In addition, whilst trauma could reduce adolescents' mental health status, it may also trigger positive changes. However, the relationship between PTSD from past trauma and posttraumatic growth is not always consistent in the literature. This might be owing to the existence of potential risk and protective factors influencing the effect of PTSD on posttraumatic growth. To advance the current research on the relation between PTSD from past trauma and specific psychological reactions, the present thesis will incorporate both positive and negative posttraumatic outcomes (PTG and psychiatric co-morbidity) in the same theoretical models. Additionally, guided by the self-trauma model (Briere & Elliott, 1994) and the models of PTG (Tedeschi & Calhoun, 2004; Calhoun & Tedeschi, 2006), the present thesis will also focus on the notions of self (trauma centrality), coping (cognitive emotion regulation), and child-caregiver relationship (unresolved attachment) and explore whether these risk and protective factors could affect the pathways between PTSD from past trauma and the two psychological outcomes.

1. 2   Overview

Following this general introduction, Chapter 2 introduces the nuanced, fine-grained inter-relationship between our main study variables, i.e., PTSD from past trauma and the positive and negative psychological outcomes characterized by posttraumatic growth and psychiatric co-morbidity. To better serve this purpose, network analysis was adopted to uncover the network structure of PTSD from past trauma, posttraumatic growth, and psychiatric co-morbidity. Chapter 3 presents the whole picture of the second study which investigated whether trauma centrality would mediate the impact of PTSD from past trauma on outcomes of posttraumatic growth and psychiatric co-morbidity. Chapter 4 introduces the third study which adopted a prospective design to verify the findings from Study Two and additionally incorporated cognitive emotion regulation to expand its results. In Chapter 5, to gain a more comprehensive view of adolescents' traumatic reactions, unresolved attachment is further integrated into Study Four to examine a theoretical framework depicting that PTSD from past trauma might co-exist with cognitive emotion regulation and unresolved attachment to influence the positive and negative psychological outcomes. Finally, Chapter 6 discusses the overall findings of the four studies and their associated implications. Suggestions for future research are also made.

Chapter 2　Study One

2.1　Introduction

2.1.1　PTSD and Posttraumatic Growth

Evidence exists to suggest that about 80% of adolescents around the world have been exposed to previous trauma, of whom 13% have experienced multiple traumas before entering adulthood (Ghazali et al., 2014; Arata et al., 2005). The prevalence rates for PTSD among adolescents can range from 22% to 51% globally (Ndetei et al., 2007; Silva et al., 2000), along with co-morbid psychiatric symptoms such as anxiety and depression (Brady et al., 2000; Armour et al., 2017; Chung et al., 2017; Chen and Chung, 2016; Chung and Chen, 2017; Wang et al., 2020). Paradoxically, the detrimental effects of trauma can motivate traumatized adolescents to experience growth (Dekel et al., 2012). They modify their disrupted core beliefs and disorganized self-schema, rebuild shattered world assumptions, and reconstruct full-functioning life (Joseph, 2012), giving rise to a new traumatized self-identity (Tedeschi and Calhoun, 1996; Boals and Schuettler, 2011). They might, as a result, improve relationships with others, develop new possibilities in life or spiritual beliefs, and enhance personal strength or appreciation of life (Tedeschi and Calhoun, 1996).

Notwithstanding this, the relationship between PTSD and posttraumatic growth (PTG) among adolescents is controversial. Although PTSD symptoms have been positively associated with PTG among adolescent survivors of various traumas (Alisic et al., 2008; Barakat et al., 2006; Hafstad et al., 2011; Kilmer and Gil-Rivas, 2010; Laufer et al., 2009; Levine et al., 2008; Du et al., 2018; Tian et al., 2016; Yu et al., 2010), this relationship has not been established among Israeli Jewish youth (Laufer et al., 2009), Chinese adolescents exposed to natural hazards (Zhou et al., 2016; Zhou et al., 2018; Yuan et al., 2018), and adolescents in the Gaza Strip (Murad and Thabet, 2017). Even when the association between PTSD and PTG was established, it might be negative (Chen et al., 2015; Wang et al., 2020) or inverted-U curvilinear (Levine et al., 2008).

Despite their inconsistency, overall these findings may corroborate previous theories of PTG suggesting that different levels of distress may be related to the development of posttraumatic growth in different ways (Butler et al., 2005; Nelson, 2011; Tedeschi & Calhoun, 2004). This makes sense, as low levels of distress are not so distressing that they challenge one's worldviews and core beliefs, and therefore may not trigger growth. High levels of distress are so overwhelming that they exceed the victims' tolerance. Therefore, victims might develop emotional numbness or cognitive and behavioral avoidance to temporarily escape trauma cues and concomitant negative affect rather than process these cues. This could undermine meaning-making and posttraumatic growth. However, in the context of moderate levels of distress, negative emotional arousal is relatively much easier to modulate and tolerate. This tolerance of distress paved the way for and set in motion subsequent cognitive processing of the trauma material, which in turn could contribute to the emergence of PTG. Nevertheless, these inconsistent results between PTSD and PTG among adolescents warrant further investigation. In particular, given the heterogeneity of PTSD (Frueh et al., 2010), how PTSD symptom clusters relate to PTG clusters remains unclear.

2. 1. 2   Psychiatric Co-morbidity and Posttraumatic Growth

Similarly, the association between co-morbid psychiatric symptoms and PTG among adolescents is also somewhat inconsistent. One study has documented a positive association between depression and PTG among Chinese adolescents who experienced natural disasters (Xu et al., 2018). This mirrors previous PTG literature indicating that the development of growth does not necessarily lead to a decrease in psychological distress. Rather,it has been observed that posttraumatic growth is often associated with some degree of distress (Tedeschi and Calhoun,1996;Tedeschi et al., 1998). This study could have reflected the illusory aspect of growth as proposed in the Janus-face model (Maercker and Zoellner, 2004). Adolescents cope with the effects of trauma by adopting unrealistic optimism and mendacious self-improvement to maintain functioning. However, because these strategies were maladaptive in nature, they could worsen psychological functioning and lead to long-term emotional problems (Zoellner and Maercker, 2006). That said, other studies observed a negative association among adolescents exposed to diverse adverse life events (Nishikawa et al., 2018;Wang et al., 2020).

2. 1. 3   Network Analysis

Existing studies exploring the interface between PTSD, psychiatric co-morbidity,and PTG mainly used the latent construct approach. However, this approach is incapable of depicting the nuanced, fine-grained inter-relationship between disorder symptoms (i.e., PTSD and co-morbid psychiatric symptoms clusters) and PTG characteristics. An alternative approach is network analysis (Epskamp et al., 2017). In contrast to the latent model, which posits that a disorder causes symptom and that these symptoms are interchangeable and equally reflective of that disorder (Cramer et al., 2010; Fried, 2015), network analysis postulates that a disorder arises from the causal interactions between symptoms. In other words, case symptoms are neither interchangeable nor reflective of that disorder (Borsboom and Cramer, 2014). For example, in terms of PTSD symptoms, reexperiencing the traumatic event might trigger negative cognitions and mood, driving avoidance and hyperarousal behaviours. These behaviours might, in turn, activate intrusion reactions (McNally et al., 2015). Such self-reinforcing loops of symptom clusters generate PTSD as a disorder (McNally, 2017).

A network consists of nodes and edges. Nodes represent symptoms, domains, or constructs (Armour et al., 2017; Jones et al., 2017a), and edges represent partial correlations between these nodes (Borsboom and Cramer, 2014). The thickness and saturation of an edge correspond to the strength of the partial correlation: the stronger the correlation, the thicker and more saturated the edge. There are two types of edges, edges within each construct and edges between constructs (i.e., bridging edges). Bridging edges connect bridging nodes across constructs. The most central nodes in a network refer to the ones within and across constructs that are highly connected and likely to drive others. Visualizing constructs in this manner sheds light on the complex interactions between them.

2.1.4 Aims

Previous studies have revealed the network structure of PTSD (e.g., concentration difficulties, detachment, irritability) and such psychiatric co-morbid symptoms as dissociation, anxiety, loss of interest, and feelings of worthlessness among clinical adults (Djelantik et al., 2019) and veterans (Armour et al., 2017). No study has thus far examined which nodes are likely to decrease (when negative bridging edges exist) or increase (when positive bridging edges exist) the co-occurrence of PTSD, psychiatric co-morbidity, and PTG (i.e. which bridging nodes of PTSD, psychiatric co-morbidity are associated with lesser or greater growth) among Chinese adolescents exposed to a past trauma. This kind of analysis may help clarify the heterogeneous relationships between the preceding constructs among adolescents and have important implications for clinical practice. The present study aimed to utilize a network analysis to 1) identify the most central nodes within each construct and the most influential bridging nodes across constructs and 2) explore bridging edges across PTSD, psychiatric co-morbidity, and PTG.

2.2   Methods

2.2.1   Participants and Procedure

Data were collected using a convenience sample. For the present study, three secondary schools (two junior middle schools and one senior high school) in a southeastern city in China were contacted. After receiving consent from the schools, the researcher (the first author) screened students from the school registers using the following inclusion criteria: 1) students who were fully enrolled in the school, 2) 13-19 years old based on Erikson's (Erikson, 1968) age range for adolescence, 3) Chinese ancestry, and 4) no special education support. The researcher went to classrooms to recruit eligible adolescents. A total of 989 students accepted the invitation, with 204 adolescents from the first grade of a junior middle school, 328 from the second and third grades of another junior middle school, and 457 from the senior high school. None declined to participate. Adolescents were explained the purpose of the study and assured of the anonymity and confidentiality of all information collected. They were then asked to complete the paper and pencil questionnaires listed in the "Measures" section in their own classrooms in one sitting. They had the right to withdraw from the study at any time without giving a reason. The adolescents gave their consent before completing the questionnaires. All the distributed questionnaires were written in Chinese and went through a back-translation procedure. The original English versions were translated into Chinese which were subsequently translated back to English by a different translator. Along with two translators, the first author of this paper scrutinized the questionnaire items where incongruence occurred until a consensus was reached. After completing the questionnaires, participants were thanked and informed that their school counsellors would be available to provide emotional support should they need. Participants were not compensated for their participation. Ethical approval was obtained from the Survey and Behavioural Research Ethics Committee at the Chinese University of Hong Kong.

Questionnaires with more than 20% missing item-level data on at least one key variable were deemed unacceptable (Parent, 2013). Accordingly, fifteen participants were excluded from the current study. In addition, of the 974 valid assessments, 11% did not report any past traumatic exposure; therefore, they were also excluded. Finally, a final sample of 867 adolescents (male=424, female=443) was included in the present study. Of them, 19% were grade 1 students from one junior middle school, 33% were grade 2 and 3 students from the other junior middle school, and 48% were senior high school students. The senior high school adolescents were older and had more psychiatric co-morbidity than the junior middle school adolescents. However, no significant differences in PTSD symptoms and posttraumatic growth were observed between these three groups of participants. They were on average 15 years old ($S=1.53$, range: 13-19), of Chinese origin, and did not attend special school. The majority of them (95%) lived in urban districts.

2.2.2   Measures

Demographic information

A demographic page was used to obtain adolescents' information on age, gender, home location, and, confirmed by the class teacher, whether they were receiving special needs education. This information aimed to assist in the selection of eligible participants.

Posttraumatic stress disorder

The Posttraumatic Stress Disorder Checklist for DSM-5 (PCL-5; Weathers et al., 2013) aims to evaluate PTSD symptoms concerning the most traumatic event. Part I asks whether adolescents were exposed to any traumatic events in the past. Those with a history of trauma were then asked to indicate the event that bothered them the most and how long ago it happened. Part II is a 20-item screening instrument (total score: 0-80) which inquiries the extent to which the participant is bothered by any PTSD symptoms in the past month using a 5-point Likert scale: 0=not at all, 1= once in a while, 2=half the time, 3=quite often, 4=always. Any item scored 2 or above would be deemed as symptomatic. The PCL-5 yields four symptom clusters: intrusion (B), avoidance (C), negative alterations in cognition and mood (D), and alterations in arousal and reactivity (E). Participants would be classified in the probable PTSD group if they reported at least one symptomatic reaction in B and C and two reactions in D and E. If only some of the four clusters met the above criteria, participants would be classified in the partial PTSD group (DSM-5; APA, 2013).

The inclusion of partial PTSD was important because partial PTSD has been frequently reported by various traumatized samples (Brancu et al., 2016; Friedman et al., 2011), including Vietnam War veterans (Weiss et al., 1992), people with eating disorders (Mitchell et al., 2012), earthquake survivors (Carmassi et al., 2013), adolescents with previous trauma (Wang et al., 2020), and first responders to the terrorist attacks in Paris (Motreff et al., 2020). Although less severe than probable PTSD, partial PTSD also affects victims' psychological functioning and is associated with a range of internalizing and externalizing problems (Marshall et al., 2001; Pietrzak et al., 2011; Zlotnick et al., 2002; Brancu et al., 2016). Identifying individuals with partial PTSD could increase knowledge about this particular group and promote effective treatment (Breslau et al., 2004; Friedman et al., 2011; Brancu et al., 2016).

The PCL-5 has been recently validated among Chinese ($\alpha = 0.93$) (Wang et al., 2020) and Malaysian adolescents ($\alpha = 0.91$) (Ghazali and Chen, 2018) and shown good psychometric properties, suggesting it is a reliable measure for the adolescent population. The Cronbach's alpha for the total score was excellent for the current study ($\alpha = 0.93$). The total scores for each of the four symptom clusters were used as nodes in the network analysis.

Psychiatric co-morbidity

The General Health Questionnaire-28 (GHQ-28; Goldberg and Hillier, 1979) aims to evaluate adolescents' probability of being diagnosed as suffering from general psychiatric disorders at an interview on a 4-point rating scale from 1 (not at all) to 4 (much more than usual). This 28-item instrument yields four dimensions: somatic symptoms, anxiety and insomnia, social dysfunction, and severe depression. The reliability coefficients of GHQ-28 ranged from 0.78 to 0.95 (Goldberg and Bridges, 1987). GHQ-28 used in previous studies to examine psychiatric symptoms among Chinese adolescents produced excellent Cronbach's alpha total scores ranging from 0.91 to 0.94 (Chen and Chung, 2016; Chung and Chen, 2017; Wang et al., 2020). For the current study, the Cronbach's alpha for the total score was excellent ($\alpha = 0.93$). The total scores for each of the four dimensions were used as nodes in the network.

Posttraumatic growth

The Posttraumatic Growth Inventory (PTGI; Tedeschi and Calhoun, 1996) estimates the perceived positive changes in the wake of the most traumatic event. The 21-item scale inquires the extent to which an individual perceives each of the 21 positive changes on a 6-point Likert scale from 0 (never) to 5 (a very great degree). The instrument produces five independent domains: relating to others, new possibilities, personal strength, spiritual change, and appreciation of life. Cronbach's alpha of this scale in a recent study among Chinese adolescents was 0.91 (Wang et al., 2020). For the current study, Cronbach's alpha for the total score was excellent ($\alpha = 0.93$). The total scores for each of the five domains were used as nodes in the network.

2.2.3　Statistical Analysis

Descriptive analyses were conducted using SPSS 25 and network analyses using different R (Version 3.6.3) packages, aiming to explore the interaction between PTSD, psychiatric co-morbidity, and posttraumatic growth. For maintaining parsimony and circumventing power problems, the domains of the three constructs rather than their original items were used in the analysis. Four primary analyses were performed: network estimation (the

R-package *qgraph*; Epskamp et al., 2012), community detection (the R-package *igraph*, Csardi and Nepusz, 2006; the R-package EGA, Golino, 2016), centrality measures (the R-package *networktools*; Jones, 2017), and accuracy and stability (the R-package *bootnet*; Epskamp et al., 2018). All visualizations were realized using the Fruchterman-Reingold algorithm (Fruchterman and Reingold, 1991) in the R-package *qgraph* (Epskamp et al., 2012).

Network estimation

We estimated the entire sample network using the Gaussian Graphical Model (GGM; Lauritzen, 1996), a network depicting the edges between nodes (four PTSD symptoms, four psychiatric co-morbid symptoms, and five PTG domains). In the GGM, edges are interpreted as partial correlation coefficients between two nodes after controlling for all other network nodes. To avoid estimating spurious edges and minimize the risk of false positives (e.g., a nonzero association is estimated although it does not exist), GGMs are estimated using the graphical least absolute shrinkage and selection operator (LASSO) (Friedman et al., 2008). The optimal model is identified using the extended Bayesian information criterion (BIC), which results in a sparse conservative and parsimonious network (Epskamp and Fried, 2018).

Community detection

Network communities are computed by assigning nodes to several sub-communities. For the current study, community detection analyses were conducted and compared using two approaches: 1) the spin glass algorithm in R-package *igraph* (Csardi and Nepusz, 2006) and 2) the Exploratory Graph Analysis (EGA) in R-package EGA (Golino, 2016). EGA produces more robust and accurate results in identifying psychometric data domains than the traditional latent factor analysis (Golino and Epskamp, 2017; Golino and Demetriou, 2017). The modularity index Q (range: 0-1) was used to quantify the strength of community structure (Newman and Girvan, 2004). The higher the Q value, the stronger the community structure. The Q value from 0.3 to 0.7 indicates a good model fit.

Centrality measures

As our network includes both positive and negative edges, the one-step expected influence (EI), rather than the commonly used centrality measures (e.g., strength, betweenness, and closeness), was preferred to identify the most central nodes within constructs (Robinaugh et al., 2016). A higher one-step EI implies a higher level of centrality in the network. Similarly, the one-step bridge expected influence (BEI) was computed to examine bridging nodes across constructs (Jones et al., 2017b). A higher one-step BEI indicates a larger bridging effect.

Accuracy and stability

The accuracy and stability analyses for the entire sample network were conducted using the recommendations from Epskamp et al. (2018). Firstly, we estimated the accuracy of network edges based on bootstrapping 95% confidence intervals (CIs) of the edge weights. The less overlap among 95% CIs, the more accurate the edge estimation. A subsequent test for edge-weight difference identified which edge significantly differed from others. Secondly, we examined the stability of centrality measures (i.e., one-step EI and one-step BEI) through case-drop bootstrapping. We also estimated the correlation stability coefficient (CS coefficient) to quantify centrality stability. The CS coefficient should be at least 0.25 for the centrality order to be considered stable, and a value above 0.5 is preferred.

2.3   Results

2.3.1   Descriptive Statistics

Regarding trauma exposure, 12% of adolescents reported one trauma and 77% reported multiple traumas. Using the Posttraumatic Stress Disorder Checklist for DSM-5, 17%, 55%, and 28% of the traumatized sample were categorized as probable PTSD, partial PTSD, and no PTSD, respectively. The most commonly reported trauma was sudden accidental death of a loved one (31%), followed by physical assault (19%), traffic accidents (16%), natural disasters (8%), and life-threatening illness or injury (8%).

2.3.2 Network Structure

All node labels, means, standard deviations, expected influences, and bridge expected influences of PTSD, psychiatric co-morbidity, and PTG domains were presented in Table 2.1.

Table 2.1 **Node labels, means, standard deviations, expected influences (EI), and bridge expected influences (BEI) for domains of PTSD, psychiatric co-morbidity, and PTG for the whole sample ($n=867$).**

Variables	Node labels for domains	μ	S	EI	BEI
PTSD	B: intrusion	5.07	4.66	1.10	0.15
	C: avoidance	1.83	2.30	0.55	0.00
	D: negative alterations in cognition and mood	5.66	5.89	1.00	0.23
	E: alterations in arousal and reactivity	4.48	4.99	0.88	0.16
Psychiatric co-morbidity	Q1: somatic symptom	13.00	4.44	0.91	0.22
	Q2: anxiety and insomnia	13.24	4.90	1.00	0.24
	Q3: social dysfunction	13.94	3.35	0.41	−0.08
	Q4: severe depression	11.07	4.46	0.70	0.14
PTG	G1: relating to others	17.69	8.49	0.72	0.00
	G2: new possibilities	12.92	6.35	1.20	−0.03
	G3: personal strength	12.03	5.07	0.96	0.00
	G4: spiritual change	3.93	2.37	0.47	0.00
	G5: appreciation of life	8.72	3.61	0.61	−0.05

The estimated domain-level network of PTSD, psychiatric co-morbidity, and PTG for the full sample was visualized in Fig. 2.1. No node was isolated in the network. Out of the 78 possible edges, 28 nonzero edges emerged, with a density of 36%. Edges within the construct were all positive, and those across constructs were both positive and negative connections. PTSD and psychiatric co-morbid symptoms and PTG domains mainly clustered within their respective constructs. Chi-square tests showed that edge densities within PTSD (83%), psychiatric co-morbidity (100%), and PTG (90%) were all significantly higher than that across PTSD and PTG (6%) (χ^2 (1) $= 17.15, p < 0.05; \chi^2$ (1) $= 26.21, p < 0.05$), across psychiatric co-morbidity and PTG (8%) (χ^2 (1) $= 20.511, p < 0.05; \chi^2$ (1) $= 23, p < 0.05$), and across PTSD and psychiatric co-morbidity (11%) (χ^2 (1) $= 10.73, p < 0.05; \chi^2$ (1) $= 15.91, p < 0.05$). These findings were corroborated by community detection analyses using spin glass algorithm and EGA, both of which identified identical three communities with substantial modularity ($Q = 0.57$), suggesting good model fit and strong community structures within the network (see Fig. S2.1).

No overlapping nodes were observed between communities. The first community included all PTSD symptom clusters, the second all psychiatric co-morbidity domains, and the third all PTG dimensions. Each community overlapped exactly with the conceptual domains of the given construct. For instance, the four nodes in the PTSD community corresponded exactly to the four DSM-5 criteria symptom clusters. These analyses supported that PTSD, psychiatric co-morbidity and PTG were distinct constructs.

Fig. 2.2 presented the standardized estimates of expected influence centrality for the whole sample network. The most central nodes within

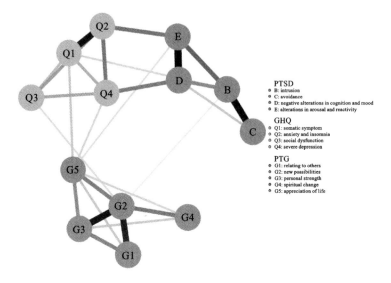

Fig. 2.1 Networks containing the domains of PTSD, psychiatric co-morbidity, and PTG for the whole sample ($n = 867$). The thickness and brightness of an edge indicate the association strength.

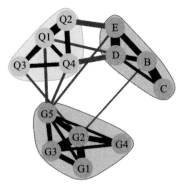

Fig. S2.1 Community analyses of the domain-level network of PTSD, psychiatric co-morbidity, and PTG for the whole sample ($n = 867$) using the spin glass algorithm and Exploratory Graph Analysis (EGA). Shaded areas indicate detected clusters. See Table 2.1 for the description of node labels.

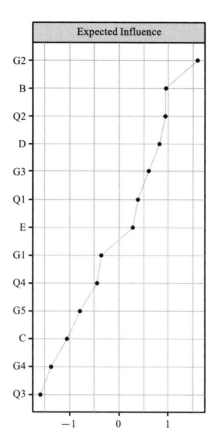

Fig. 2.2　**Standardized expected influence centrality indices for domains of PTSD,**
psychiatric co-morbidity, and PTG for the whole sample ($n=867$). See Table
2.1 for the description of node labels.

constructs were intrusion (B) for PTSD, anxiety and insomnia (Q2) for
psychiatric co-morbidity, and new possibilities (G2) for PTG (see Fig. 2.2
and Fig. S2.2). As the network included both positive and negative bridging
edges, there were positive and negative BEI values for bridging nodes, with
positive BEI values indicating positive cross-community influences and
negative values implying negative impacts (see Fig. 2.3 and Fig. S2.3). The
most influential bridging node for PTSD symptom clusters was negative
alterations in cognition and mood (D), for psychiatric co-morbidity domains

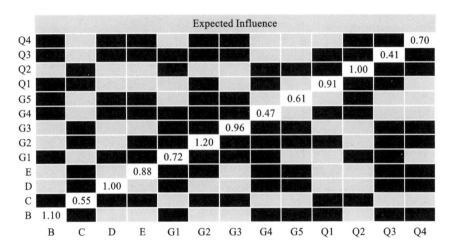

Fig. S2.2 **Bootstrapped difference tests ($\alpha = 0.05$) between the expected influence of PTSD, psychiatric co-morbidity, and PTG domains for the whole sample ($n = 867$). Gray boxes indicate nodes that do not differ significantly from one another and black boxes represent nodes that do differ significantly from one another. White boxes show the value of node strength. See Table 2.1 for the description of node labels.**

was anxiety and insomnia (Q2), and for PTG dimensions was appreciation of life (G5). The case-drop bootstrap indicated that the order of EI and BEI was stable enough for interpretation with a CS coefficient being 0.75 and 0.36, respectively.

The edge weights bootstrap (see Fig. S2.4) showed that the domain-level network of PTSD, psychiatric co-morbidity, and PTG was moderately accurately estimated. Eight bridging edges emerged across constructs, with two across PTSD and PTG (one positive, intrusion with new possibilities (B-G2), and one negative, alterations in arousal with appreciation of life (E-G5)), three across psychiatric co-morbidity and PTG (one positive, somatic symptom with appreciation of life (Q1-G5), and two negative, social dysfunction with new possibilities (Q3-G2) and severe depression with appreciation of life (Q4-G5)), and three across PTSD and psychiatric co-

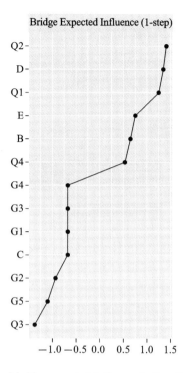

Fig. 2.3   Standardized bridge expected influence indices for domains of PTSD,

psychiatric co-morbidity, and PTG for the whole sample ($n = 867$).

See Table 2.1 for the description of node labels.

morbidity (all positive, negative alterations in cognition and mood with somatic symptom (D-Q1), negative alterations in cognition and mood with severe depression (D-Q4), alterations in arousal and reactivity with anxiety and insomnia (E-Q2)) (see Fig. 2.1).

Proportional chi-square tests revealed no significant differences in edge densities between the three cross-communities (i.e., the PTSD-psychiatric co-morbidity community, the PTSD-PTG community, and the psychiatric co-morbidity-PTG community) (χ^2 (1) $=0.09, p>0.05; \chi^2$ (1) $=0, p>0.05;$ $\chi^2(1)=0, p>0.05$). Among the eight bridging edges, alterations in arousal and reactivity with anxiety and insomnia (E-Q2) and alterations in negative cognition and mood with severe depression (D-Q4) were the strongest. The

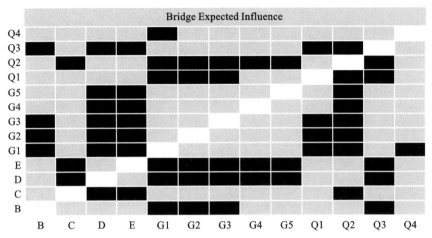

Fig. S2.3   Bootstrapped difference tests ($\alpha = 0.05$) between the bridge expected influence
of PTSD, psychiatric co-morbidity, and PTG domains for the whole sample ($n =$
867). Gray boxes indicate nodes that do not differ significantly from one another
and black boxes represent nodes that do differ significantly from one another.
See Table 2.1 for the description of node labels.

• Bootstrap mean   • Sample

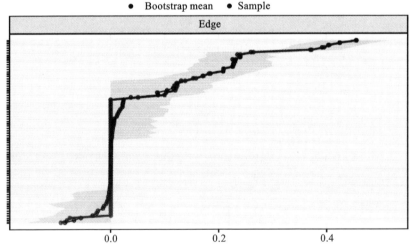

Fig. S2.4   Bootstrapped confidence intervals of estimated edge weights for the estimated
domain-level network of PTSD, psychiatric co-morbidity, and PTG for the
whole sample ($n = 867$). The gray line indicates the sample values and the
gray area the bootstrapped CIs. Each horizontal line represents one edge of
the network, ordered from the edge with the highest edge weight to the edge
with the lowest edge weight.

remaining six were comparable to each other (see Fig. S2.5). Moderate overlap among the bootstrap 95% CIs of edge weights suggested that the order of bridging edges should be interpreted with some care.

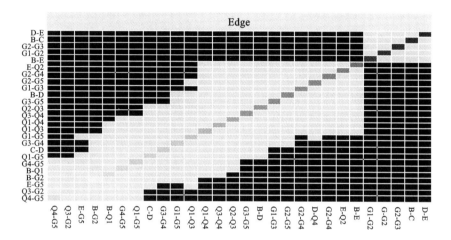

Fig. S2.5 Bootstrapped difference tests ($\alpha=0.05$) between edge weights that were nonzero in the estimated domain-level network of PTSD, psychiatric co-morbidity, and PTG for the whole sample ($n=867$). Gray boxes indicate edges that do not differ significantly from one another and black boxes represent edges that do differ significantly from one another. See Table 2.1 for the description of node labels.

2.4 Discussion

To the best of our knowledge, the current study was the first to explore the network structure of PTSD, psychiatric co-morbidity, and PTG among Chinese adolescents. The domains of these psychological constructs mainly clustered in their respective communities, within which edges were all positive. The most central nodes were intrusion (B), anxiety and insomnia (Q2), and new possibilities (G2) for PTSD, psychiatric co-morbidity, and PTG, respectively. Intrusion (B) being the most central node within PTSD echoed prior studies arguing that over and above other symptoms, it played a critical role in the development and persistence of PTSD (Cao et al., 2019; Russell et al., 2017; Bartels et al., 2019; De Haan et al., 2020; Ge et al., 2019). Although, on average, the onset of the traumatic event was 17 months ago (S=27.3), over 60% of the sample still had repeated, disturbed, and unwanted memories of the trauma; 68% felt upset when they were reminded of the event; 52% felt they relived the experience. The severity of intrusion symptoms seemed to persist over time (Nijdam et al., 2013).

In terms of anxiety and insomnia, 76% of adolescents reported that they constantly felt under strain; over half (58%) felt nervous, strung up, edgy all the time, and had a bad temper; 46% to 49% had problems with sleep due to worry and stress. Aside from the effects of their traumatic experiences, anxiety and insomnia could also be related to the academic stress and interpersonal stress these adolescents felt. Academic stress and interpersonal stress were common among adolescents in China (Sun, 2012; Cohen et al., 2013; Fan et al., 2016), which were consistently associated with mental health problems such as anxiety, depression, and sleeping difficulties (Zakari et al., 2008; Sun, 2012; Fuligni et al., 2009; Cohen et al., 2013; Gunn et al., 2014). For new possibilities (G2) to be the most central node for PTG echoed the literature (e.g., Bellet et al., 2018) focusing on bereaved university students. The majority (91%) of the adolescents reported that they felt able to do better things and change what needed changing in their lives; 80% were able to develop new interests, and 68% found new opportunities, which was thought to be the main essence of growth (Robinaugh and McNally, 2013; Nerken, 1993).

The present results identified positive and negative bridging edges across three constructs. After controlling for all the other nodes in the network, the intrusion (B) cluster showed a positive association with new possibilities (G2) and somatic symptom (Q1) with appreciation of life (G5). These findings were in line with previous studies on a positive relationship between psychological symptoms and PTG among adolescents (Xu et al., 2018). Specifically, the association between intrusion (B) and new possibilities (G2) echoed the literature on victims exposed to various traumas (Alisic et al., 2008; Barakat et al., 2006; Hafstad et al., 2011; Kilmer and Gil-Rivas,2010; Laufer et al., 2009; Levine et al., 2008; Du et al., 2018; Tian et al., 2016; Yu et al., 2010) and a claim from a meta-analysis that increased intrusion is associated with increased growth (Helgeson et al., 2006).

The intrusive memories caused by intrusion symptoms might constantly remind victims of their unprocessed trauma and concomitant schema incompatibility (Horowitz, 1980; Berntsen and Rubin, 2006). According to the "completion principle" (Horowitz, 1982), they at the same time have a tendency to assimilate the existing schema with the traumatized one and integrate trauma into their autobiographical memory system, which is likely to set in motion, in PTG terms, the constructive processing of unresolved materials (Calhoun and Tedeschi, 2006). This process is a cognitive one that is associated with deliberate and reflective ruminations aimed at making sense of trauma (Cann et al., 2010; Joseph and Linley, 2004). A better understanding of trauma could in turn facilitate misbelief abandonment, schema revision, and meaning-making required by the development of posttraumatic growth (Tedeschi et al., 2018; Tedeschi and Calhoun, 2004). This experience of personal growth might further produce a positive affect. Adolescents might have therefore become motivated to find new possibilities in life as was depicted earlier (Boals and Schuettler, 2011; Joseph, 2012; Robinaugh and McNally, 2013; Calhoun and Tedeschi , 2006), appreciate their daily life (91%), cherish their own life (89%), and reorder life priorities

(77%), despite the physical discomfort from somatic symptoms.

However, two bridging nodes of psychiatric co-morbidity were related to the weakening of the PTG community: social dysfunction and new possibilities (Q3-G2) and severe depression and appreciation of life (Q4-G5). Depression seldom correlates positively with posttraumatic growth. Instead, it is often negatively correlated with growth. This observation is not surprising, given that depression is usually associated with negative thinking, which makes it difficult to perceive any positive aspects of a situation, let alone a traumatic one (LaRocca and Avery, 2020; Zoellner and Maercker, 2006). The present study added to the literature by pointing specifically towards the difficulty in appreciating their life in general. Also, since social dysfunction is a constituent of depression and can be disabling in managing daily tasks, enjoying normal daily activities, and making decisions, it is not surprising that victims found it challenging to search for new possibilities. This finding is concordant with prior findings of a negative association between psychiatric co-morbidity and PTG (Nishikawa et al., 2018; Wang et al., 2020).

The present results seemed to have contradicted the youth resilience hypothesis (Masten, 2014). While some adolescents can rise above extremely difficult conditions and long-term health issues and strive for resilience, some might have restricted resilience ability and cast doubt on the emergence of a "survivorship" identity (Abernathy, 2008; Sadler-Gerhardt et al., 2010). Their ability to accept and appraise their vulnerability and develop a renewed appreciation for life seemed to have been restricted (Abernathy, 2008; Neimeyer, 2006; Sadler-Gerhardt et al., 2010). The current results have also echoed that mental health symptoms can be a barrier to posttraumatic growth. Instead, trauma victims tend to create negative cognitions, restrict their ability to make meaning out of the situation (LaRocca and Avery, 2020;

Mazor et al., 2016), and make it difficult for authentic positive changes like new opportunities and appreciation towards life to emerge (Maercker and Zoellner, 2004).

It has been argued that psychological symptoms are accompanied by cognitive-affective disturbances giving rise to negative appraisal or anticipation, enhancing pain catastrophizing and negative emotions (Mostafaei et al., 2019). Those with psychiatric co-morbidities also tend to have high levels of neuroticism and introversion (Menon et al., 2018). These cognitive-affective disturbances, along with the personality traits mentioned above, could have reduced adolescents' likelihood of appreciating life and seeing new possibilities.

In addition to these cognitive-affective disturbances, according to the impaired disengaged hypothesis (Koster et al., 2011), whilst it is natural to ruminate on some negative trauma-related issues to make sense of the event or our personal history (Carver and Scheier, 1998), some trauma victims (adolescents in this case) might have difficulty in exercising attentional control. They are unable to disengage attention from negative affect elicitors and distress-specific stimuli. Their preoccupation would only lead to maladaptive rumination in maintaining negative affect or hopelessness (Ciesla and Roberts, 2007; Nolen-Hoeksema, 1991), which could reduce the likelihood of seeing new possibilities and appreciating their current life.

Concerning the findings on the association between PTSD and psychiatric co-morbidity, whilst they stood as two distinct communities in the network, the bridging edges between their respective communities were all positive. This finding echoes the claim that PTSD is not a discrete syndrome, but is expressed through psychiatric co-morbid symptoms (Miller et al., 2003; Miller et al., 2004). The current results suggested an association between alterations in arousal and reactivity and anxiety and insomnia (E-

Q2). This observation accords with previous network studies focusing on diverse traumatized adult samples (Armour et al., 2017; Afzali et al., 2017; Choi et al., 2017). The connection between alterations in arousal and reactivity and anxiety and insomnia might be accounted for by their overlapping symptoms of difficulty relaxing, sleep problems, and irritability (Afzali et al., 2017; Choi et al., 2017).

The current results also identified the association between negative alterations in cognition and mood and severe depression (D-Q4), which is in line with prior findings (Armour et al., 2017; Afzali et al., 2017; Djelantik et al., 2019). These results are not surprising given that depression and negative alterations in cognitions and mood often share similar psychological issues around feelings, mood, and self-worth (Djelantik et al., 2019). The above association may be particularly striking in the context of trauma. Traumatized victims tend to perceive the world as unsafe, others as untrustworthy, and themselves as unlovable (Janoff-Bulman, 1989). They may even blame themselves or others for the event. These distorted cognitions can interfere with normal psychological functioning, intensify existing distress, induce negative feelings of hopelessness and helplessness, and generate mistaken beliefs of worthlessness (Briere and Elliott, 1994). However, such negative feelings and mistaken beliefs were the fundamental constituents of depression (Beck, 1996). Depression, as mentioned earlier, was associated with negative thinking patterns and excessive emotional distress. When these distressing emotions exceeded the victim's tolerance, emotional numbness or cognitive avoidance symptoms were likely to occur (Briere, 1996; Horowitz, 1976), preventing unresolved issues from being processed or understood (Tedeschi and Calhoun, 2004). In addition, the negative thinking patterns associated with depression disrupt attention deployment and immerse victims in the negative context of trauma (Koster et al., 2011). This would inhibit the constructive processing of trauma cues (Tedeschi and Calhoun, 2004; Calhoun and Tedeschi, 2006). As a result, victims were unable to make sense of the trauma and make sense of life (Zoellner and Maercker, 2006), which in turn could affect the way they value their own lives, set life priorities, and appreciate each day (Q4-G5).

Also, our study observed a significant connection between intrusion and somatic symptom (B-Q1). This finding might reflect a "conversion" phenomenon. Adolescents' past traumatic effects can be experienced on a sensory level as "body memories" (Briere, 2002; Gupta et al., 2005; van der Kolk and Fisler, 1995) and manifest themselves as unexplained somatic complaints. In other words, these adolescents could have converted their traumatic intrusive memories into more acceptable somatic complaints (Engel, 2004; Gupta, 2006; Gupta et al., 2005). For instance, the disturbing and unwanted memories of the trauma repeatedly intrude on the victim's consciousness, which can lead to strong physical reactions such as palpitations and difficulty breathing, as well as negative feelings such as agitation and anxiety. These physical and emotional reactions are stressful to the body and can increase the physiological work of the autonomic nervous system (Lahav et al., 2016), leading to an escalation of somatic problems, making victims feel unwell.

Somatic complaints, in turn, appeared to increase life appraisal, as shown previously (Q1-G5). This is at odds with a meta-analysis which claimed that poor subjective health was not related to posttraumatic growth (Helgeson et al. , 2006). While PTG may be related to different types of psychological symptom clusters, physical health, and quality of life (Helgeson et al., 2006), a psychological symptom cluster could also be related to a specific type of growth. This finding is consistent with the cognitive content-specific hypothesis (Beck et al., 1976), which states that affective states can be distinguished by unique cognitive content. Somatization-related affects (e.g., headache or exhaustion) could be associated with specific cognitive thoughts of adolescents. Their thought content could have specific implications for how they appraise their current lives. For example, distress caused by somatic pain could elicit anxiety-related thoughts related to death, which in turn could cause victims to value their own lives more. The illness could also cause them to reconsider what is truly important to them and reorder priorities in life. The current finding also mirrors previous evidence of a positive association between posttraumatic growth and somatic complaints (Lahav et al., 2016) or psychiatric distress (Xu et al., 2018; Calhoun and Tedeschi, 2006).

There were several limitations to Study 1. Firstly, our sample could have been biased. Participants were recruited from three secondary schools located in the same district of the city out of convenience. They were not, therefore, a representative sample which calls for caution with the generalizability of findings. Additionally, our sample was nonclinical. This status could have distorted the strength and number of associations between constructs (Afzali et al., 2017). Secondly, this was a cross-sectional study that did not identify a causal relationship between nodes. A longitudinal design would have been needed (Bringmann et al., 2015). Nonetheless, our findings of bridging edges could help understand the structural relationships between PTSD, psychiatric co-morbidity, and PTG, despite the lack of causality inference (Holland, 1986). Thirdly, the current study did not consider the impact of cultural characteristics on the network structures. The Chinese collectivist culture in which these adolescents were raised emphasizes harmonious relationships with others, interdependence with family or community members, and social obligations (Jayawickreme et al., 2013; Oyserman and Lee, 2008). The comfort and support provided by family and community members in this culture might buffer the pathogenic effects of trauma and promote recovery (Wright et al., 2013). In addition, cultural differences have been shown to influence the growth experiences of individuals (Waugh et al., 2018). Therefore, the educational culture of these adolescents may have influenced the number and strength of connections between constructs.

To conclude, whether adolescents with a history of past trauma appreciate life or perceive new possibilities in the future would depend on a mixture of trauma-specific and general psychological distress reactions. These might shed some light on the facilitation of patients' posttraumatic growth by clinical psychiatrists.

Chapter 3   Study Two

3. 1   Introduction

3. 1. 1   PTSD, Trauma Centrality, and Psychiatric Co-morbidity

To recap, disputes over the relationship between PTSD and posttraumatic growth were noted among previous samples of traumatized adolescents. Despite these inconsistencies, there are theoretical postulates suggesting that PTSD could impact posttraumatic growth and psychiatric co-morbidity indirectly through mediating variables. Given that adolescents are at the crucial stage for identity formation (Erickson, 1968) and their cognitive capacities are under-developed (Briere, 1992), the cognitive schema of this population might be particularly vulnerable in the presence of overwhelming trauma. Accordingly, trauma centrality, a concept targeting identity and self-schema, was postulated to be one of these mediating variables in the current study.

Trauma centrality is used to depict the fact that trauma can have a detrimental impact on the concept of self (Wilson, 2006) and can give rise to a drastic re-evaluation of oneself. The vividness of traumatic memories can enter victims' awareness and drive them to appraise the traumatic event as central to their lives (Conway & Pleydell-Pearce, 2000). They then overestimate the frequency of traumatic events, increase hypervigilance and avoidance behavior and thereby increase the likelihood for re-traumatization. These memories form personal reference points from which victims attribute meaning to current beliefs, feelings, and future expectations. Their outlook on life and life course are consequently affected and redirected. These traumatic memories and profound changes in the sufferers themselves have become turning points in their lives, reconfigured their inner worlds and re-defined their personal identities (Fitzgerald, 1988; Berntsen & Rubin, 2006; Pillemer, 2003).

Trauma centrality is essentially a form of posttraumatic cognitive schema incompatible with existing schema. According to the "completion principle" advocated in the Stress Response Syndrome (Horowitz, 1980, 1982, 1983), victims try to revise, accommodate, and assimilate the internal trauma psychic model with existing schema. Such incompatibility and the process of assimilation heighten levels of psychiatric co-morbid symptoms (Janoff-Bulman, 1992). Thus, it is not surprising that adolescents with PTSD reported a significantly higher level of trauma centrality than their counterparts (Ionio et al., 2018). Trauma centrality was also associated with psychiatric distress including depression, anxiety, and other co-morbid symptoms among college students (Boals & Schuettler, 2011; Groleau et al., 2013; Barton et al., 2013; Wamser-Nanney et al., 2018), sexually abused women (Robinaugh & McNally, 2011), and refugees (Chung et al., 2017, 2018).

3. 1. 2   Trauma Centrality and Posttraumatic Growth

Notwithstanding this, trauma centrality, like a double-edged sword (Boals & Schuettler, 2011), could also relate to posttraumatic growth in the aftermath of trauma. Guided by previous PTG theories, posttraumatic growth could emerge from experiences that are significant enough (i.e., central) to challenge one's core beliefs and basic assumptions (Janoff-Bulman,1992), and would develop after the integration of trauma into one's autobiographical memory system (Tedeschi & Calhoun, 2004; Tedeschi et al., 2007). Construing an event as central to one's identity and life narrative implies that the core beliefs have been challenged and modified, worldviews have been re-examined and altered, and more importantly, life narratives have been re-organized and continued via the reconciliation of trauma with personal identity (Berntsen & Rubin, 2006; Boals & Schuettler, 2011). Also, the highly vivid and accessible memories caused by trauma centrality could play some part in the developmental course of PTG (Fitzgerald et al., 2016; Lancaster et al., 2015). In other words, these memories might constantly remind victims of their unprocessed trauma and concomitant schema incompatibility (Berntsen & Rubin, 2006). According to the "completion principle" (Horowitz, 1982), they at the same time have a tendency to assimilate the existing schema with the traumatized one and integrate the crisis into their autobiographical memories, which is likely to set in motion, in PTG terms, the constructive processing of unresolved materials (Calhoun & Tedeschi,2006). This process is a cognitive one that enables victims to make sense of trauma and establish meaning, as a result of which personal growth is enhanced.

Not surprisingly, trauma centrality was observed in relation to escalated posttraumatic growth among university students and adult survivors even after controlling for depression, dissociation, neuroticism, previous PTSD, coping strategies, and demographic variables (Schuettler & Boals, 2011; Boals & Schuettler,2011; Groleau et al., 2013; Brooks et al., 2017; Wamser-Nanney et al., 2018). However, three other studies of trauma centrality reported mixed results regarding these two constructs. Whilst trauma centrality was positively associated with PTG among a sample of undergraduates, no significant relation was observed within the sample of treatment-seeking women (Barton et al., 2013). Similarly, in a large-scale investigation across 10 countries, although trauma centrality was related to increased posttraumatic growth among adults and undergraduates from all 10 countries, this was not replicated when looking at participants from each country separately (Taku et al., 2021). Specifically, samples from Australia, Germany, Poland, and Turkey perceiving the event as central to their identity and life story, also reported higher levels of posttraumatic growth, but for those from the other six countries (i.e., Italy, Japan, Nepal, Peru, Portugal, and the US), trauma centrality did not affect the development of posttraumatic growth. Moreover, evidence from a longitudinal study, based on employees in the Norwegian ministries who were exposed to the 2011 Oslo bombing, supported a concurrent relation but not a longitudinal one between trauma centrality and PTG (Blix et al., 2015). In other words, whilst trauma centrality and posttraumatic growth were concurrently positively associated with each other at both 10 and 22 months following the bombing, earlier trauma centrality did not predict subsequent growth. Nonetheless, to the best of our knowledge, no studies have investigated the relationship between trauma centrality and posttraumatic growth among adolescents.

3.1.3   Aims and Hypotheses

What has been described is a hypothesized model depicting the inter-relationship between PTSD from past trauma, trauma centrality, psychiatric co-morbidity, and posttraumatic growth (see Fig. 3.1). No studies thus far have examined this model among Chinese adolescents, and the aim of Study 2 was to do so. In testing this model, potential confounding factors need to be taken into account. Firstly, academic stress is particularly prominent among adolescents in China and East Asia (Sun, 2012). Indeed, it was a strong predictor of depression and school burnout (Sun, 2012; Yan et al., 2018). Similar results were found among adolescents in other countries. For example, academic stress was positively associated with burnout among French adolescents (Walburg et al., 2014; Zakari et al., 2008) and with social withdrawal, depression, anxiety, and somatic problems among Latino adolescents (Torres & DeCarlo Santiago. ,2017), as well as with depression among Hispanic (Cervantes et al., 2015), Korean (Lee, 2016), and Singaporean (Ang & Huan, 2006) adolescents. Secondly, adolescents' demographic information also needs to be considered since several studies have highlighted the fact that "victim variables" can impact PTSD severity and psychiatric co-morbid symptoms (Friedman et al., 2007; Vogt et al. , 2007). After controlling for academic stress and demographic variables, we hypothesized that 1) PTSD would be positively associated with posttraumatic growth, trauma centrality, and psychiatric co-morbidity and 2) trauma centrality would mediate the impacts of PTSD on posttraumatic growth and psychiatric co-morbidity.

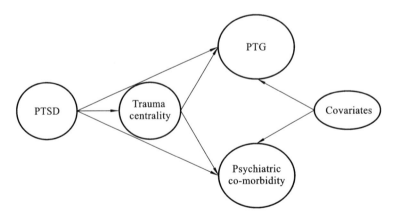

Fig. 3.1 **The hypothesized model for Study 2 with covariates (demographic information and academic stress) adjusted for.**

3. 2   Methods

3. 2. 1   Participants and Procedure

Data was collected using a convenience sampling method. Two high schools located in a metropolitan city in China were contacted for the study. After obtaining permission from the schools, the researcher asked eight teachers (who taught courses to different classes in Grade 1) to assist in identifying qualified participants from the classes they were teaching. In case students were distressed when responding to certain questionnaire items, the researcher also invited the psychology teachers (who had previously received professional training in Psychological First Aid) at these two schools to provide relevant counselling services.

The inclusion criteria for participants of the present study were as follows: (1) senior high school students in Grade 1 (i.e., students who were 15 years old and above and were first-year students of high school), (2) of Chinese ethnicity, and (3) no special needs education received according to school records with confirmation from the head teacher. Subsequently, nine hundred and sixty-two senior high school adolescents in Grade 1 were invited to participate in the study, and all of them accepted. Participants were met in their respective classrooms by the researcher during the class times of the eight teachers. The aim of the study was explained to the participants who were then asked to complete the questionnaires listed in the "Measures" section in class. The adolescents were ensured that all information collected would be kept anonymous and strictly confidential and that they had the right to withdraw from the study at any time without giving a reason. All adolescents provided consent before participation and after the data collection, they were thanked and informed that their psychology teachers at school were available to provide support (e.g., group counselling), should they wish to receive treatment following the study.

Fourteen students left most parts of the questionnaires unanswered; therefore, they were excluded from the final analysis. All the distributed questionnaires were in Chinese and went through the same back-translation procedure as elucidated in Study 1. Ethical approval was then obtained from the Survey and Behavioral Research Ethics Committee at the Chinese University of Hong Kong.

Nine hundred and forty-eight adolescents (male = 462, female = 486) participated in the study. On average, they were 15 years old ($S = 0.54$, range= 14-17), of Chinese ethnicity, students in their first year of high school, and receiving no special needs education.

3.2.2　Measures

Demographic information

A demographic page was used to obtain the adolescents' information regarding age, academic year, gender (0 = female, 1 = male), and, with confirmation from the head teacher, whether they were receiving special needs education. This information was used to assist with the selection of students.

Posttraumatic stress disorder

The Posttraumatic Stress Disorder Checklist for DSM-5 (PCL-5; Weathers et al., 2013) aims to assess PTSD symptoms related to past trauma. Part I focuses on a list of traumatic events that adolescents have previously experienced. If they have experienced more than one trauma, adolescents are asked to indicate the trauma that bothers them the most and how long ago it happened. Part II is a screening instrument used to evaluate

PTSD symptoms with the most traumatic event as the index trauma using the rating scale:0=not at all,1=once a week or less/once in a while,2=two to three times a week/half of the time,3=four or five times a week/quite often,4=six or seven times a week/always. The PCL-5 has shown good agreement and reliability with the Structured Clinical Interview for Diagnosis (kappa=0. 65, agreement=82%, sensitivity=0. 89, specificity=0. 75). This scale consists of four symptom clusters:intrusion (B) (e. g., Repeated, disturbing and unwanted memories of the stressful experience?), avoidance (C) (Avoiding memories, thoughts, or feelings related to the stressful experience?), negative alterations in cognition and mood (D) (Blaming yourself or someone else for the stressful experience or what happened after it?),and alterations in arousal and reactivity (E) (Feeling jumpy or easily startled?). When the questionnaire items are scored 2 or above, they are considered as symptomatic. Using the DSM-5 diagnostic criteria,meeting the criteria for probable PTSD would require adolescents to have at least one symptomatic response in B and C symptom clusters as well as two symptomatic responses in D and E. If the number of symptomatic responses is less than the responses required for some of the symptom clusters, they would be classified as meeting the diagnostic criteria for partial PTSD. If the number of symptomatic responses is less than what is required for all symptom clusters, they would be classified as having no PTSD. The PCL-5 was validated among Malaysian adolescents (α=0.91) (Ghazali & Chen, 2018;Murphy et al.,2018) and Chinese adolescents (α=0.91,0.94,and 0.93, respectively) (Liu et al., 2016; Yang et al., 2017), and revealed good psychometric properties, suggesting that it is a reliable measure for adolescents. Based on the current sample, the Cronbach's alpha scores for the total score was 0.93.

Psychiatric co-morbidity

The General Health Questionnaire-28 (GHQ-28; Goldberg & Hillier,

1979) estimates the probability for adolescents to be diagnosed as suffering from general psychiatric disorders at interview using a rating scale from 1 (not at all) to 4 (much more than usual). It includes four subscales: somatic problems (e.g., Been feeling perfectly well and in good health?), anxiety (Had difficulty in staying asleep once you are off?), social dysfunction (Been managing to keep yourself busy and occupied?), and depression (Been thinking of yourself as a worthless person?). And reliability coefficients ranged between 0.78 and 0.95 (Goldberg & Bridges, 1987). GHQ-28 was used in previous studies to examine psychiatric symptoms among Chinese adolescents with Cronbach's alpha scores reaching 0.91 and 0.94 for the total score (Chen & Chung, 2016; Chung & Chen, 2017). For the current sample, the Cronbach's alpha for total score was 0.94.

Posttraumatic growth

The Posttraumatic Growth Inventory (PTGI; Tedeschi & Calhoun, 1996) assesses perceived positive life changes as a result of a traumatic event. The 21 items are rated on a 6-point scale ranging from 0 (never) to 5 (a very great degree), with higher scores indicating greater PTG. The scale yields five independent factors: strengthening of social relationships (e.g., I have a greater sense of closeness with others.), new possibilities (I developed new interests.), perception of personal resources and skills (I know better that I can handle difficulties.), spiritual change (I have a stronger religious faith.), and appreciation of life (I can better appreciate each day.). The Cronbach's alpha of this scale in a recent study based on Chinese adolescents was 0.94 (Yuan et al., 2018). For this study, the Cronbach's alpha for the total score was 0.91.

Trauma centrality

The Centrality of Events Scale (CES; Berntsen & Rubin, 2006) is a 20-item questionnaire measuring to what degree the traumatic event has become

(a) a reference point for everyday inferences (e.g., This event has become a reference point for the way I understand new experiences.), (b) a central part of an adolescent's personal identity (I feel that this event has become part of my identity.), and (c) a turning point in an adolescent's life story (This event is making my life different from the life of most other people.). Items are rated on a 5-point scale, ranging from 1 (totally disagree) to 5 (totally agree), and summed to yield a total score. This scale has been validated in studies based on Portuguese adolescents (α for total score = 0.95; α for the 3 subscales = 0.87, 0.89, and 0.85, respectively) (Cunha et al., 2015; Vagos et al., 2018) and Italian adolescents (α for the 3 subscales = 0.85, 0.82, and 0.86, respectively) (Ionio et al., 2018), and has achieved good test-retest reliability, and concurrent, convergent, and discriminant validity, suggesting that CES is a reliable measure for adolescents with diverse ethnicities. For the current sample, the Cronbach's alpha for the total score was 0.94.

Academic stress

The Educational Stress Scale for Adolescents (ESSA; Sun et al., 2011) measures adolescents' academic stress on five aspects: pressure from study (e.g., I feel a lot of pressure in my daily studying.), workload (I feel there is too much homework.), worry about grades (I feel that I have disappointed my parents when my test/exam results are poor.), self-expectation (I feel stressed when I do not live up to my own standards.), and despondency (I always lack confidence with my academic scores.). The scoring is based on a 5-point Likert scale ranging from 1 (strongly disagree) to 5 (strongly agree), with a higher total score indicating a higher level of academic stress. This scale has shown good consistency, reliability, concurrent validity, and a Cronbach's alpha of 0.81 for the total score. For the current sample, the Cronbach's alpha was 0.88 for the total score.

3. 2. 3   Statistical Analysis

Statistical analysis was conducted using SPSS 25 and Mplus 7. 4. Initial analysis was carried out using descriptive statistics, Pearson's correlation, and multivariate analyses of variances (MANOVA) with Bonferroni correction to minimize the likelihood of type I error. MANOVA aimed to compare differences between probable PTSD, partial PTSD, and no PTSD groups in trauma centrality, posttraumatic growth, and psychiatric co-morbidity. We also estimated effect sizes using partial eta-squared statistics and evaluated them based on Cohen's suggestion (1988), with 0.01-0.058 being small, 0.059-0.137 being medium, and 0.138 and above being large.

Structural equation modeling (SEM) was used to test the hypothesized mediation model with adjusted demographic variables and academic stress. In addition, Maximum likelihood (ML) was adopted to estimate parameters. ML has shown to be robust and accurate even with moderately and extremely skewed data (Hau & Marsh, 2004). Similarly, Finney and DiStefano (2006) proposed that SEM behaves rather well when the absolute value of skewness and kurtosis for latent variables are below 2 and 7 respectively. In the current study, the absolute values of skewness and kurtosis for all latent variables ranged from 0.17 to 0.98, indicating that although the data was skewed, ML was the proper fit function for parameter estimation.

Good model fit indices were adopted to evaluate the hypothesized model: a root mean square error of approximation (RMSEA) below 0.08, a comparative fit index (CFI) above 0.90, a non-normed fit index (NNFI/TLI) above 0.90, and a standardized root mean square residual (SRMR) below 0.06 (McDonald & Ho, 2002). The Chi-square test was not used as indices because the χ^2 value is almost always statistically significant for models with a moderate or large sample size.

3.3   Results

3.3.1   Descriptive Statistics and Correlation

All means, standard deviations, and correlations between variables are depicted in Table 3.1. Using the PCL-5, 34% of adolescents did not report any trauma. On the other hand, 28% experienced one trauma whilst 38% experienced multiple traumas; 18%, 58%, and 24% of the traumatized adolescent sample met the DSM-5 screening criteria for probable PTSD, partial PTSD, and no PTSD, respectively. The most frequently reported trauma was physical assault (40%), followed by serious accident (13%), natural disaster (11%), life-threatening illness or injury (10%), and childhood abuse (5%). The average onset of the most traumatic event was 3.63 (S=3.07) years ago.

Prior to the SEM analysis, Pearson correlations were carried out to establish whether demographic variables and academic stress were related to psychological outcomes (psychiatric co-morbidity and posttraumatic growth). If so, they were controlled for in the SEM analysis. Moreover, ethnicity, age, academic year, and whether the adolescents were receiving special education were not included in the correlation analysis since all participants were Chinese, more or less the same age, in the same academic year, and not receiving any special education. Gender was the only demographic variable entered into the correlation. The results showed that females were more likely to demonstrate co-morbidity symptoms than males; academic stress was positively correlated with psychiatric co-morbidity and negatively associated with posttraumatic growth (see Table 3.1).

Table 3.1　Means, standard deviations, and Pearson correlations between variables ($n=948$).

Variables	1	2	3	4	5	6	7
1. Gender[①]	1						
2. Age	0.159 **	1					
3. Academic stress	−0.056	−0.001	1				
4. PTSD	−0.035	−0.035	0.456 **	1			
5. Trauma centrality	0.062	−0.019	0.346 **	0.617 **	1		
6. PTG	0.062	0.001	−0.152 **	−0.102 **	0.115 **	1	
7. Psychiatric co-morbidity	−0.108 **	−0.012	0.555 **	0.624 **	0.379 **	−0.277 **	1
μ	−	15.28	54.50	18.54	50.54	60.84	53.34
S	−	0.542	10.62	15.690	17.487	17.302	14.435

Note: ① point biserial correlation (r_{pb}), dummy variables: 0=female; 1=male.

** $p<0.01$.

3.3.2　Multivariate Test between Diagnostic Groups

Multivariate analyses of variances showed that there were significant differences between three diagnostic groups in trauma centrality, posttraumatic growth, and psychiatric co-morbidity. To wit, the probable PTSD group reported significantly higher levels of trauma centrality and psychiatric co-morbidity than the partial PTSD group (centrality: 95% CI= 12.34 to 17.53; co-morbidity: 95% CI=12.25 to 16.60) and the no PTSD group (centrality: 95% CI=25.28 to 31.25; co-morbidity: 95% CI=19.74 to 24.75). In contrast, the probable PTSD group reported significantly lower levels of posttraumatic growth than the other two groups (partial PTSD: 95% CI=−8.35 to −2.38; no PTSD: 95% CI=−7.65 to −0.79) (see Table 3.2).

Table 3. 2　Means and standard deviations of trauma centrality, PTG, and psychiatric co-morbidity between diagnostic groups ($n=948$).

	Probable PTSD μ (S)	Partial PTSD μ (S)	No PTSD μ (S)	F	Post hoc analyses $p<0.05$	Partial η^2
Trauma centrality	66.07 (13.51)	51.14 (15.18)	37.80 (15.45)	173.54	Probable>Partial>No	0.269
Psychiatric co-morbidity	67.13 (14.47)	52.70 (12.69)	44.88 (10.54)	153.63	Probable>Partial>No	0.245
PTG	56.70 (15.74)	62.07 (15.56)	60.92 (21.45)	6.23	Probable<Partial=No	0.013

3.3.3　Measurement Model

Before examining the hypothesized model, SEM examined the measurement model and showed that the loadings of the indicators of the four latent constructs (PTSD, PTG, trauma centrality, and psychiatric co-morbidity) were significantly different from zero (see Table 3.3).

Table 3.3　Standardized factor loadings for the measurement model ($n=948$).

Latent variable	Indicator	B	S. E.	P
PTSD				
	Intrusion	0.789	0.019	0.000
	Avoidance	0.617	0.027	0.000
	Negative alterations	0.853	0.015	0.000
	Alterations in reactivity	0.842	0.015	0.000
Trauma centrality				
	Reference point	0.917	0.009	0.000
	Central to identity	0.895	0.010	0.000
	Turning point	0.805	0.014	0.000

Continue

Latent variable	Indicator	B	S. E.	P
PTG				
	Relation to others	0.723	0.021	0.000
	New possibilities	0.900	0.012	0.000
	Personal strength	0.810	0.017	0.000
	Spiritual change	0.538	0.026	0.000
	Appreciation of life	0.757	0.020	0.000
Psychiatric co-morbidity				
	Somatic problems	0.737	0.019	0.000
	Anxiety	0.857	0.014	0.000
	Social dysfunction	0.661	0.023	0.000
	Depression	0.778	0.019	0.000

3.3.4　Structural Model

The hypothesized mediation model was then examined using SEM with gender and academic stress controlled for. Standardized regression coefficients, standard errors, and residual variances for all paths and indicators are presented in Fig. 3.2. The results showed a good model fit (χ^2 = 1042.387, df = 220, χ^2/df = 4.738, RMSEA = 0.063, CFI = 0.926, TLI = 0.916, SRMR = 0.053). They also demonstrate that posttraumatic stress disorder from past trauma was positively associated with trauma centrality (β = 0.684, p < 0.001, 95% CI = 0.636 to 0.730) and psychiatric co-morbidity (β = 0.596, p < 0.001, 95% CI = 0.493 to 0.697), but negatively associated with posttraumatic growth (β = -0.305, p < 0.001, 95% CI = -0.447 to -0.178). In addition, trauma centrality was positively related to posttraumatic growth (β = 0.446, p < 0.001, 95% CI = 0.338 to 0.536), but negatively related to psychiatric co-morbidity (β = -0.126, p < 0.01, 95% CI

$=-0.204$ to -0.046). Finally, trauma centrality significantly mediated the paths between PTSD and PTG (the indirect effect $=0.305$, $p<0.001$, 95% CI$=0.228$ to 0.371), as well as between PTSD and psychiatric co-morbidity (the indirect effect $=-0.086$, $p<0.01$, 95% CI$= -0.143$ to -0.032).

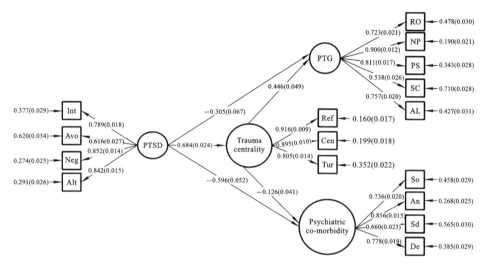

Fig. 3.2   **Model test result for Study 2 with standard beta weights, standard error, and residuals added ($n=948$). This model took account of the covariates of gender and academic stress. All the paths were significant. See List of Abbreviations for the full names of variables and indicators.**

3.4   Discussion

The current study investigated the relationship between PTSD, trauma centrality, posttraumatic growth, and psychiatric co-morbidity among Chinese adolescents. Contrary to hypothesis 1, with gender and the level of academic stress adjusted, whilst PTSD was positively associated with psychiatric co-morbidity and trauma centrality, it was negatively associated with posttraumatic growth. Consistent with hypothesis 2, trauma centrality significantly mediated the impacts of PTSD on posttraumatic growth and psychiatric co-morbidity.

The prevalence rate (18%) for probable PTSD among our adolescents in the current study was compatible with the 19% reported in the literature also focusing on traumatized adolescents in China (Chen & Chung, 2016). Indeed, in line with previous findings (Chen & Chung, 2016; Chung & Chen, 2017; Yang et al., 2017; Xu et al., 2018; An et al., 2019), adolescents with PTSD reported elevated psychiatric co-morbidity. This result is not surprising given that PTSD is not a concrete clinical syndrome but often co-exists with and expresses itself through other psychological disorders (Chung et al., 2017; Miller et al., 2004; Keane et al., 2007).

PTSD from past trauma was negatively associated with posttraumatic growth among our adolescent sample, which contradicted some literature focused on youth (Alisic et al., 2008; Barakat et al., 2006; Hafstad et al., 2011; Kilmer & Gil-Rivas, 2010; Kilmer et al., 2009; Laufer & Solomon, 2006; Laufer et al., 2009; Levine et al., 2008; Yu et al., 2010; Zhou et al., 2015; Tian et al., 2016; Vloet et al., 2014; Yuan et al., 2018), but echoed other literature (Du et al., 2018). In light of the Janus-face model (Maercker & Zoellner, 2004), PTG has two components, self-deceptive illusory growth and self-transforming authentic growth. The illusory component, characterized by deceiving oneself with unrealistic optimism and mendacious self-enhancement, often occurs and accumulates shortly after a crisis as a temporary defense against immediate distress. The authentic component, in contrast, functions as an adaptive strategy to cope with the detrimental effects of trauma, i.e., activating the constructive processing of trauma cues to promote self-transcendence. As the process of self-transformation usually takes time, the concomitant self-transformative growth also develops and accumulates long after a crisis. Not surprisingly, self-deceptive illusory growth is related to avoidance behaviors, denial, and worse psychological functioning such as heightened PTSD, depression, and anxiety, whereas self-transforming authentic growth is associated with improved psychological well-being in the aftermath of trauma (Maercker & Zoellner, 2004).

Arguably, our finding might reflect the one aspect of the Janus-face model which suggests that growth is perhaps an illusory self-deceptive concept. Despite the fact that the most traumatic event happened nearly four years ago, these victims still coped with the effect of trauma by adopting unrealistic optimism toward their future (Maercker & Zoellner, 2004), thereby leading to reduced likelihood for authentic constructive growth to emerge. Additionally, according to the impaired disengagement hypothesis (Koster et al., 2011), as a result of the trauma, adolescents might have found themselves experiencing negative thoughts and moods and developing negative self-relevant beliefs that led to difficulty in shifting attention from the negative perception to making meaning from the trauma. Such difficulty would hamper the process of posttraumatic growth, since meaning-making is an important constituent for it (Tedeschi & Calhoun, 2004).

Notwithstanding this, taking account of trauma centrality, a different picture emerged. Although the traumatic event happened, on average, almost 4 years ago, the link between PTSD and trauma centrality was still relevant to these adolescents at the time of the study, echoing literature that focused on college students (Schuettler & Boals, 2011; Boals & Schuettler, 2011; Barton et al., 2013; Groleau et al., 2013; Wamser-Nanney et al., 2018). According to mediation results, traumatized adolescents who reported a high level of trauma centrality increased posttraumatic growth and improved psychological well-being. In other words, those who reported profound changes in re-organizing self-structure and identity, and viewing current and future experiences, the world, as well as their life stories tended to display the constructive self-transforming aspect of growth that promotes functional adaptation and adjustment after the trauma (Maercker & Zoellner, 2004).

In line with the adversarial growth thesis, although trauma might have affected the self-concept of these adolescents, which in turn triggered their tendency to facilitate this growth process as a coping process (Joseph & Linley, 2004), they engaged in some cognitive processes which enabled them to modify their worldview, develop a new self-structure focused on developing a new identity, outlook on life, and attribution to meanings to current and future experience (Boals & Schuettler, 2011; Chen et al., 2015; Berntsen & Rubin, 2006; Tedeschi & Calhoun, 1996; Tedeschi et al., 2007), and reducing positive illusions while enhancing existential matters (Creamer et al., 1992; Greenberg, 1995). These processes were associated with an increase in the constructive or adaptive aspect of posttraumatic growth (Zoellner & Maercker, 2006) which buffered against or mitigated distress from trauma (Taylor & Armor, 1996; Chen et al., 2015). According to the positive youth literature (Masten, 2014), their resilience process could have been strengthened by the meaning-making process, i.e., making sense of their trauma experience and integrating trauma memories into their personal identities which, in turn, would help in their trauma recovery. This has been the case for some adolescents despite the sensitive developmental changes that they have gone through (Vagos et al., 2018).

Possibly, the adolescents' Chinese cultural upbringing had an impact on the development of their resilience. Indeed, it has been postulated that resilience is often rooted in culture, especially ones in which community and family support, security, or comfort in relating to community members may buffer against the impact of traumatic experiences (Wright et al., 2013). The collectivist culture, of which the current sample was a part, emphasizes the importance of interdependent, familial, harmonious relationships and mutual or social obligation within the community (Jayawickreme et al., 2013;

Oyserman & Lee, 2008) as possibly contributing to the level of resilience. However, systematic research is needed to examine whether collectivism or individualism or familism for that matter might relate to elevated protection or resilience (Gaines et al., 1997).

There were limitations in Study 2. Firstly, our sample might have been biased since the two secondary schools in our study were located in the same district of the city. Also, only the adolescents in Grade 1 were included in the study; therefore, the generalizability of the findings is called into question. Secondly, this was a cross-sectional study which restricted our interpretation of the mediation results in terms of causal relationships due to the lack of temporal precedence (Cole & Maxwell, 2003). Notwithstanding this, the mediation results could be used to attempt to understand the structural relationship of the model without drawing causality inference (Holland, 1986). Finally, no information was collected on the degree of identity consolidation among these adolescents. To what extent they developed a sense of continuity with past experiences, present meanings, and future direction was unknown (Marcia, 1994). This information could have influenced distress outcomes or growth.

To conclude, around seventy percent of the adolescents recruited for the study were exposed to one or more traumatic events in the past. Their traumas influenced the way they perceived the benefits of their traumatic experiences and the severity of their general psychological distress. Prima facie, PTSD from past trauma was associated with reduced posttraumatic growth and elevated psychological distress. These trauma responses were in fact dependent on whether PTSD had changed the way adolescents viewed their daily experience, expected from future experience, and restructured their personal identity.

Chapter 4　Study Three

4.1　Introduction

To recap, in Study 2, after controlling for gender and academic stress, PTSD from past trauma positively predicted psychiatric co-morbidity and trauma centrality but negatively predicted posttraumatic growth. In addition, trauma centrality significantly mediated the impacts of PTSD on posttraumatic growth and psychiatric co-morbidity. However, as pointed out in the limitations section of Study 2, the cross-sectional nature of the study limited our interpretation of the causal relationships between constructs, due to the lack of temporal precedence (Cole & Maxwell, 2003). Hence, to verify the mediational results of Study 2, a longitudinal approach was proposed for Study 3.

4.1.1　PTSD and Cognitive Emotion Regulation

Additionally, findings of Study 1 suggest that traumatized adolescents with high levels of trauma centrality experienced more personal growth and better psychological well-being, which points to the resilience of adolescents. This might be related to the certain types of coping tactics that traumatized youths employ to regulate distressing affects (Wang et al., 2020). As argued by the stress response syndromes (Horowitz, 1976) and the self-trauma model (Briere, 1992), trauma shatters the way victims perceive the self, others, and the world and gives rise to a traumatized identity incompatible with the existing schema, whereby a discrepancy could induce tremendous psychological distress. To prevent themselves from being overwhelmed and to protect themselves, victims may engage in certain coping strategies to modulate the intense emotions to a tolerable extent (Briere, 1992; Schimmenti & Caretti, 2016; Thomson & Jaque, 2018; Slanbekova et al., 2019). Cognitive emotion regulation (CER) could be postulated as one of these coping strategies. To understand more about the role of this coping tactic in posttraumatic adjustment, the current longitudinal study also explores the function of cognitive emotion regulation in responding to trauma.

Before looking at cognitive emotion regulation, it is worth pointing out that most current coping measures incorporate the cognitive and behavioral approaches in the same dimension, including emotion-focused coping strategies of denial (cognitive) and social support seeking (behavioral), and problem-focused coping strategies of planning (cognitive) and taking direct actions (behavioral) (Garnefski et al., 2001). This is deemed inappropriate as thinking (cognitive) and acting (behavior) represent two distinct processes (Garnefski et al., 2001). Apart from cases of conditioned and unconditioned reflexes, thinking, under most circumstances, tends to precede acting and affect subsequent behaviors. Also, actions following constructive cognitions are more adaptive and fruitful in responding to crises. Hence, to assist victims in taking appropriate actions when dealing with distress, it would be more meaningful to first teach them the cognitions behind these actions (Garnefski et al., 2001). As such, victims learn the mechanisms associated with constructive actions and are therefore able to modify their own actions according to cognitions in the context of new challenges so that these problems could be better addressed. Cognitive emotion regulation was born in the context of this argument and highlights the importance of cognitions or cognitive processes in managing negative emotional arousals from catastrophic events, i.e., what victims think (rather than what they do) regarding the crisis (Garnefski et al., 2001; Thompson, 1991). These cognitions can be functional or dysfunctional, giving rise to two broad types of cognitive emotion regulation, i.e., adaptive cognitive emotion regulation (adaptive CER) and maladaptive cognitive emotion regulation (maladaptive CER) (Garnefski et al., 2001).

Maladaptive CER is characterized by negative strategies of exaggerating the terror of trauma (catastrophizing), blaming oneself (self-blame) or blaming others (other blame) for the event, and focusing one's attention and thoughts on the negative context of crisis (rumination). Therefore, it is not surprising to find Ugandan and Israeli adolescents with PTSD also reporting escalated maladaptive CER strategies of rumination and other blame (Amone-P'Olak et al., 2007; Pat-Horenczyk et al., 2014). By contrast, adaptive CER refers to positive strategies of thinking about something pleasant rather than the traumatic condition (positive refocusing), resigning oneself to the highly stressful event (acceptance), degrading its severity (putting into perspective), figuring out what steps can be taken to improve the situation (refocusing on planning), and attaching a positive meaning to it (positive reappraisal). However, findings on the relationship between PTSD and adaptive CER were inconsistent among adolescents. Whilst PTSD was negatively associated with adaptive CER strategies of refocusing on planning and putting into perspective among Ugandan adolescents (Amone-P'Olak et al., 2007), no significant relation could be established among Israeli youths (Pat-Horenczyk et al., 2014). Given this inconsistency of findings and the cross-sectional nature of past research on the association between PTSD and cognitive emotion regulation among adolescents, further investigation with a prospective design might be more appropriate to address these issues.

4. 1. 2   Cognitive Emotion Regulation and Psychiatric Co-morbidity

Since coping strategies (in this case, cognitive emotion regulation) employed to confront trauma may in turn shape psychological outcomes (Aldao et al., 2010), it is reasonable to assume that the two types of cognitive emotion regulation (adaptive CER and maladaptive CER) might mediate the impact of PTSD from past trauma onto psychiatric co-morbidity. In particular, previous cross-sectional evidence among university students suggests a significant mediation of self-blame (a maladaptive CER strategy) on the relation between PTSD and psychiatric co-morbidity (Slanbekova et al., 2019). Nonetheless, it is unclear whether the mediational mechanisms of adaptive CER and maladaptive CER are tenable among adolescents.

The relationship between the two types of cognitive emotion regulation and psychiatric co-morbid symptoms is well-established in the literature. Adaptive CER reflects more efficient coping and functions to mitigate psychological distress and contributes to posttraumatic adaptation following adversity (Garnefski et al., 2001; Garnefski et al., 2008). Increasing evidence from preceding studies has supported that engagement in adaptive CER strategies (e. g., positive reappraisal, positive refocusing, refocusing on planning, and acceptance) was related to less endorsement of depression, anxiety, and other internalizing problems among Eastern and Western adolescents (Garnefski et al., 2001; Garnefski & Kraaij, 2006; Stikkelbroek et al. , 2016; Amone-P'Olak et al., 2007; d'Acremont & Van der Linden, 2007; Li et al., 2015; Rey Peña & Extremera Pacheco, 2012; Madjar et al., 2019). Nevertheless, all these studies were cross-sectional except for Li et al. (2015) which found that initial positive reappraisal predicted reduced depression one year later. This paucity of longitudinal literature on the relationship between adaptive CER and psychiatric co-morbidity calls for attention from researchers.

Contrastingly, maladaptive CER implies deficits in cognitive emotion regulation and tends to exacerbate psychological suffering and hamper posttraumatic recovery (Aldao et al., 2010; Garnefski et al., 2001; Garnefski et al., 2008). Therefore, it is reasonable to find that traumatized adolescents resorting to maladaptive cognitive emotion regulation strategies (e. g., self-blame, rumination, and catastrophizing) suffered increased general psychological symptoms including depression and anxiety (Amone-P'Olak et al., 2007; d'Acremont & Van der Linden, 2007; Auerbach et al., 2010; Li et al., 2015; Rey Peña & Extremera Pacheco, 2012; Madjar et al., 2019; Pat-Horenczyk et al., 2013; Garnefski et al., 2001; Garnefski & Kraaij, 2006; Stikkelbroek et al., 2016). Nonetheless, as illustrated previously, among all of these studies, only one was prospective and demonstrated a significant prediction of initial rumination and catastrophizing on escalated depression one year later (Li et al., 2015). Longitudinal evidence on the relationship between maladaptive CER and psychiatric co-morbid symptoms was limited.

4.1.3 Cognitive Emotion Regulation and Posttraumatic Growth

Likewise, cognitive emotion regulation can also mediate the effects of PTSD from past trauma on posttraumatic growth. Guided by the PTG literature (Tedeschi & Calhoun, 2004), trauma does not naturally trigger personal growth; the key to turning posttraumatic suffering into posttraumatic growth lies in the ability to reconcile trauma with victims' schema and rebuild a self-structure that can operate in the posttraumatic world. These abilities, however, place heavy demands on the processes of affect regulation and cognitive readjustment. The former (affect regulation) serves to regulate and reduce emotional distress within tolerable levels, so as to set in motion the latter (cognitive readjustment) that facilitates decentering from the pathogenic effects of trauma onto the positive context of crisis and initiates the constructive processing of traumatic cues. Together, these cognitive emotion regulation processes could enhance understanding of crisis, assimilate the stressful experience into personal identity, and establish meaningfulness in life, thereby contributing to the formation of posttraumatic growth (Calhoun & Tedeschi, 2006). Given that individual differences in transformative coping against trauma could impact adaptation outcomes (Aldwin et al., 1994), adaptive CER and maladaptive CER, differing in adaptivity, may exert different mediational effects on the relation between PTSD and posttraumatic growth.

Notwithstanding this, the relationship between the two types of cognitive emotion regulation and PTG has been under-investigated among adolescents. Indeed, preliminary evidence regarding these two constructs has predominantly emerged from adults. For instance, among college students (Hanley et al., 2017; Thomas et al., 2019), bereaved adults (Aguirre, 2008), patients with myocardial infarction (Garnefski et al., 2008), and adult patients with multiple sclerosis (Aflakseir & Manafi, 2018), adaptive CER strategies (e.g., positive refocusing, positive reappraisal, and acceptance) were found to be associated with higher levels of posttraumatic growth even after controlling for meaning-making and purpose in life. By contrast, maladaptive cognitive emotion regulation strategies were not related to the development of PTG (Aguirre, 2008; Garnefski et al., 2008; Aflakseir & Manafi, 2018). Nevertheless, to what extent adaptive CER and maladaptive CER are associated with posttraumatic growth among adolescents remains to be uncovered.

4.1.4 Aims and Hypotheses

Focusing on a group of Chinese adolescents with past trauma, this 6-month follow-up investigation aimed to explore 1) the relationship between baseline PTSD and two psychological outcomes, i.e., psychiatric co-morbidity and posttraumatic growth at T3 (6-month follow-up), and 2) whether trauma centrality, adaptive CER, and maladaptive CER at T2 (3-month follow-up) would respectively mediate the impacts of baseline PTSD on these two psychological outcomes at T3.

Similar to Study 2, in examining the hypothesized model, several potential confounding factors were taken into account. Firstly, academic stress, which is particularly prominent among adolescents in China and East Asia (Sun, 2012) and is related to depression, anxiety, burnout, social withdrawal, somatic problems and posttraumatic growth among Eastern and Western adolescents (Sun, 2012; Wang et al., 2020; Walburg et al., 2014; Zakari et al., 2008; Torres & DeCarlo Santiago, 2017; Cervantes et al., 2015; Lee, 2016). Secondly, initial psychiatric co-morbidity, initial PTG, and PTSD at T3 also needed to be controlled for. Psychological distress, such as depression or anxiety, is a chronic mental health issue (Russel et al., 2001), which might linger on and accumulate stress to affect later distress and growth outcomes. Also, this distress outcome tends to have an enduring connection with PTSD (Miller et al., 2004; Keane et al., 2007). Posttraumatic growth can be a continuous type of phenomenon, exerting a long-lasting influence on subsequent growth and psychological well-being (Tedeschi & Calhoun, 2004). Finally, adolescents' demographic information can influence outcomes, as "victim variables" can affect the severity of PTSD and psychiatric co-morbid symptoms (Friedman et al., 2007; Vogt et al.,

2007). After controlling for demographic variables, academic stress, psychiatric co-morbidity at baseline, baseline PTG, and PTSD at T3, we hypothesized as follows (see Fig 4.1).

1) Baseline PTSD would be positively associated with psychiatric co-morbidity and PTG at T3.

2) Baseline PTSD would be positively associated with trauma centrality at T2 which would, in turn, be positively associated with psychiatric co-morbidity and PTG at T3; trauma centrality at T2 would mediate the impact of baseline PTSD on these two psychological outcomes at T3.

3) Baseline PTSD would be positively related to adaptive CER at T2 which would, in turn, be negatively related to psychiatric co-morbidity at T3 but positively related to PTG at T3; adaptive CER at T2 would mediate the effect of baseline PTSD on these two psychological outcomes at T3;

4) Baseline PTSD would be positively related to maladaptive CER at T2 which would, in turn, be positively related to psychiatric co-morbidity at T3 but negatively related to PTG at T3; maladaptive CER at T2 would mediate the impact of baseline PTSD on these two psychological outcomes at T3.

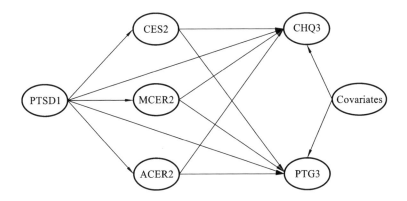

Fig. 4.1   The hypothesized model for study three.

4. 2　Methods

4. 2. 1　Participants and Procedure

One junior high school and one senior high school located in a metropolitan city in China were contacted for the current study. After providing detailed explanations regarding the purpose and procedures of the study to the school principals, permission for data collection was obtained. The two psychology teachers and five course teachers at these schools selected the classes they were teaching for the researcher who then identified qualified students to participate. Similar to Study 2, these psychology teachers were invited to provide counselling support to participants throughout the study. The inclusion criteria for participants were as follows: 1) of Chinese ethnicity, and 2) registered in the participating schools, as confirmed by the school records. As with Study 2, participants were met in their respective classrooms by the researcher during the course time of the aforementioned seven teachers. Following a full description of the study with an emphasis on anonymity, confidentiality and voluntary participation, students were asked to provide consent and then complete a battery of self-report questionnaires (see the "Measures" section) in class. Likewise, after each wave of data collection, adolescents were thanked and informed that they could turn to their psychology teacher at school for counselling support should they need it. All the distributed questionnaires were in Chinese and went through the same back-translation procedure as elucidated in Study 1. Ethical approval was obtained from the Survey and Behavioral Research Ethics Committee at the Chinese University of Hong Kong.

This study was divided into three waves with a time interval of 3 months. The initial assessment recruited eight hundred and ninety-six adolescents to complete measures of demographic information, academic stress, PTSD, psychiatric co-morbidity, and PTG (T1). None of them opted out. As the current study would only include participants with traumatic experiences in the past, those not reporting any prior trauma were excluded, leaving 802 adolescents eligible for wave 1. To facilitate the subsequent follow-up, the participant's date of birth, the kin type of their primary caregiver (e.g., father, mother, grandmother, or grandfather), and the last four numbers of the primary caregiver's cellphone number were used to track students over time, given the anonymity of self-report questionnaires. The second wave was conducted three months following baseline assessment and included 778 of the original 802 participants (T2, response rate=97.0%) to complete measures of trauma centrality and cognitive emotion regulation. The third wave took place six months after baseline assessment and included 765 of the original 802 students (T3, response rate=95.4%; the attrition rate between T1 and T3=4.6%) to complete measures of PTSD, psychiatric co-morbidity, and PTG. The attrition rate resulted from some students transferring to other schools and others dropping out. The current study only included participants who completed valid assessments at all three waves; therefore, those who were absent from any subsequent participation and/or submitted invalid assessments were excluded from final analysis.

A final sample of seven hundred and fifty-seven adolescents ($n=757$; male=400, female=357) participated in the three-wave longitudinal study. On average, they were 15 years old ($\mu=14.80, S=1.19$, range=12-19) and all of Chinese ethnicity.

4. 2. 2 **Measures**

Demographic information

The same demographic page of Study 2 was adopted in Study 3 but with participants' birthdays, the kin types of their primary caregiver (e.g., father, mother, grandmother, or grandfather), and the last four numbers of the primary caregiver's cellphone number added. This additional information was aimed at following up with the students.

Posttraumatic stress disorder, Psychiatric co-morbidity, Posttraumatic growth, and Academic stress

For the measurement of these constructs, the same instruments as described in Study 2 were adopted in Study 3. Based on the current sample, the Cronbach's alpha scores for the total score of PTSD were 0.94 (T1) and 0.96 (T3); for the total score of psychiatric co-morbidity, they were 0.94 (T1) and 0.94 (T3); for the total score of PTG, they were 0.93 (T1) and 0.96 (T3); and for the total score of academic stress, it was 0.89 (T1).

Trauma centrality

To avoid overwhelming students with a large number of questionnaire items, the short form of the Centrality of Events Scale (The 7-item CES; Berntsen & Rubin, 2006) was adopted by the current study. Based on the current sample, the Cronbach's alpha for the total score was 0.91 (T2).

Cognitive emotion regulation

The Cognitive Emotion Regulation Questionnaire-Short (CERQ-short; Garnefski & Kraaij, 2006) measures what adolescents think in responding to a traumatic event. Adolescents rate each of the 18 items from 1 (almost never) to 5 (almost always). The CERQ-short generates nine conceptually distinct cognitive emotion regulation strategies, with five being adaptive/ positive (acceptance (e.g., I think that I have to accept that this has happened.), positive refocusing (I think of something nice instead of what has happened.), refocusing on planning (I think about a plan of what I can do best.), positive reappraisal (I think I can learn something from the situation.), and putting into perspective (I tell myself that there are worse things in life.)) and four being maladaptive/negative (self-blame (I think that basically the cause must lie within myself.), rumination (I often think about how I feel about what I have experienced.), catastrophizing (I continually think how horrible the situation has been.), and blaming others (I feel that basically the cause lies with others.)). Subscale scores are obtained by summing the items under this subscale with higher subscale scores indicating more salient use of this specific strategy. The CERQ-short has shown good psychometric properties with Cronbach's alphas for subscales ranging from 0.62 to 0.85 (Garnefski & Kraaij, 2006), and has been reliably validated among Spanish adolescents (Rey Peña & Extremera Pacheco, 2012) and Israeli adolescents (Madjar et al., 2019). Based on the current sample, the Cronbach's alpha scores for adaptive cognitive emotion regulation and maladaptive cognitive emotion regulation were 0.87 (T2) and 0.83 (T2), respectively.

4. 2. 3   Statistical Analysis

Initial descriptive analyses, including descriptive statistics, Pearson's correlations between measured constructs, and case summaries were conducted using SPSS 25. Subsequently, structural equation modeling (SEM) was conducted using Mplus 7.4. Prior to testing the hypothesized mediation model, we first examined the measurement model of latent variables: PTSD at T1, trauma centrality, adaptive CER and maladaptive CER at T2, and psychiatric co-morbidity and PTG at T3. Next, with demographic variables, academic stress, baseline psychiatric co-morbidity, baseline posttraumatic growth, and PTSD at T3 controlled, we tested the hypothesized mediation model, including direct paths from initial PTSD to psychiatric co-morbidity and PTG at T3 and indirect links from initial PTSD to these two psychological outcomes at T3 via mediators (i.e., trauma centrality, adaptive CER, and maladaptive CER at T2). Finally, for sub-analyses, we also examined the above hypothesized mediation model by excluding academic stress, initial psychiatric co-morbidity, and PTSD at T3 from the covariates (i.e., we controlled only for demographic variables and baseline PTG). Bias-corrected bootstrap tests ($n = 1000$) with a 95% confidence interval were then conducted to examine the indirect mediation effects (Gootzeit & Markon, 2011). Maximum likelihood (ML), which performed robustly and accurately even with skewed data, was finally employed to estimate parameters (Hau & Marsh, 2004).

In addition, the following model fit indices were adopted to evaluate the measurement and hypothesized model: a comparative fit index (CFI) and a non-normed fit index (NNFI/TLI) equal to or greater than 0.90, a root mean square error of approximation (RMSEA) less than 0.08 (McDonald & Ho, 2002), and a standardized root mean square residual (SRMR) below 0.08 (Wen et al., 2004). The Chi-square (χ^2) test was not used as model fit indices in the current study since it is nearly always statistically significant under a moderate or large sample size.

4.3 Results

4.3.1 Descriptive Statistics and Correlation

All means, standard deviations, and correlations between study variables are presented in Table 4.1. Using the PCL-5, 15% of the traumatized adolescents encountered one trauma, and 85% suffered multiple traumas. The most frequently reported event was traffic accident (72%), followed by sudden death of someone close (64%), life-threatening illness or injury (46%), and natural disaster (32%). The average onset of the most stressful experience was 4.35 ($S=3.53$) years ago. At baseline, 18%, 44% and 38% of the traumatized adolescent samples met the DSM-5 screening criteria for probable PTSD, partial PTSD, and no PTSD, respectively. Six months later, the prevalence rates for probable PTSD, partial PTSD, and no PTSD became 19%, 38%, and 43%, respectively. Further analysis of case summaries revealed that 52% of adolescents had no change in PTSD diagnostic status from baseline to 6-month follow-up, 13% showed delayed onset of PTSD, and 9% deteriorated to probable PTSD. On the other hand, 7% and 19% of the adolescents experienced partial and full recovery of PTSD, respectively, after six months.

Prior to SEM analysis, Pearson correlations were conducted to examine whether demographic variables, academic stress, initial psychiatric co-morbidity, initial PTG, and PTSD at T3 were associated with posttraumatic outcomes (i.e., psychiatric co-morbidity and PTG at T3). If so, they were adjusted in the SEM analysis. As our adolescents did not differ in ethnicity (i.e., all were Chinese), only age, gender, academic stress, initial psychiatric co-morbidity, initial PTG, and PTSD at T3 were then entered into the correlation. Findings indicated that being older, female, and under higher pressure of academic stress was associated with greater severities of psychiatric co-morbidity and lower levels of posttraumatic growth at T3. Initial psychiatric co-morbidity and initial PTG were related to the two psychological outcomes at T3. PTSD at T3 was positively associated with psychiatric co-morbidity at T3 but not related to PTG at T3. (see Table 4.1).

Table 4.1 Means, standard deviations, and correlations between variables ($n=757$).

Variables	$\mu \pm S$	1	2	3	4	5	6	7	8	9	10	11	12
1. Gender	—	1											
2. Age	14.80±1.19	-0.066	1										
3. Academic stress	51.70±12.21	0.004	0.326**	1									
4. GHQ1	49.64±14.51	0.157**	0.209**	0.549**	1								
5. PTG1	54.60±22.59	-0.051	-0.107**	-0.099**	-0.232**	1							
6. PTSD1	17.18±16.69	0.069	0.034	0.401**	0.655**	0.002	1						
7. PTSD3	17.24±17.72	0.100**	0.018	0.303**	0.481**	-0.032	0.589**	1					
8. MCER2	19.29±7.00	-0.118**	0.105**	0.273**	0.343**	0.062	0.420**	0.418**	1				
9. ACER2	30.01±9.16	-0.062	0.038	0.037	0.019	0.249**	0.121**	0.092*	0.580**	1			
10. CES2	17.40±7.22	-0.103**	-0.024	0.220**	0.279**	0.078*	0.423**	0.362**	0.501**	0.237*	1		
11. GHQ3	51.24±15.67	0.146**	0.215**	0.398**	0.561**	-0.226**	0.407**	0.630**	0.302**	-0.001	0.221**	1	
12. PTG3	50.27±27.66	-0.100**	-140**	-0.087*	-0.188**	0.458**	0.012	-0.007	0.079*	0.270**	0.093*	-0.277**	1

Note: See List of Abbreviations for the description of variables. 0=male; 1=female.

* $p<0.05$, ** $p<0.01$.

4. 3. 2   Measurement Model and Structural Model

The measurement model using SEM exhibited good fit indices ($\chi^2 =$ 1 271. 377, df$=260$, χ^2/df$=4.89$, RMSEA$=0.072$, CFI$=0.920$, TLI$=$ 0. 907, SRMR$=0.065$) with factor loadings of all latent variables (PTSD at T1, trauma centrality, adaptive CER and maladaptive CER at T2, and psychiatric co-morbidity and PTG at T3) significantly different from zero. However, subsequent examination of the structural model displayed a poor model fit. Inspections on modification indices (MI) suggested that adding the covariate between maladaptive CER and adaptive CER at T2 should greatly improve the model fit. Hence, we added a covariate path between these two constructs accordingly (see Fig. 4. 2). The final structural model (with age, gender, academic stress, initial psychiatric co-morbidity, initial PTG, and PTSD at T3 adjusted for) was examined again and produced a good model fit ($\chi^2 =2$ 140. 327, df$=561$, χ^2/df$=3.82$, RMSEA$=0.061$, CFI$=0.912$, TLI $=0.902$, SRMR$=0.081$) (see Fig. 4.2).

Standardized regression coefficients and standard error for all pathways are presented in Fig. 4.2. Baseline PTSD was positively associated with trauma centrality at T2 ($\beta=0.480$, $p<0.001$, 95% CI$=0.404$ to 0. 542), adaptive CER at T2 ($\beta=0.149$, $p<0.001$, 95% CI$=0.078$ to 0. 235), maladaptive CER at T2 ($\beta=0.486$, $p<0.001$, 95% CI$=0.411$ to 0. 562), and PTG at T3 ($\beta=0.189$, $p<0.05$, 95% CI$=0.027$ to 0. 368), but negatively associated with psychiatric co-morbidity at T3 ($\beta=-0.263$, $p<0.01$, 95% CI$=-0.418$ to -0.100). Trauma centrality at T2 was not associated with psychiatric co-morbidity at T3 ($\beta=0.014$, $p>0.05$, 95% CI $=-0.053$ to 0.091) or PTG at T3 ($\beta=0.032$, $p>0.05$, 95% CI$=-0.058$ to 0.124). Adaptive CER at T2 was not related to psychiatric co-morbidity at

T3 ($\beta = -0.127$, $p > 0.05$, 95% CI $= -0.329$ to 0.080) but positively related to PTG at T3 ($\beta = 0.486$, $p < 0.01$, 95% CI $= 0.255$ to 0.854). Maladaptive CER at T2 was not associated with psychiatric co-morbidity at T3 ($\beta = 0.138$, $p > 0.05$, 95% CI $= -0.083$ to 0.384) but negatively associated with PTG at T3 ($\beta = -0.361$, $p < 0.05$, 95% CI $= -0.784$ to -0.072). In addition, maladaptive CER and adaptive CER at T2 were positively correlated with each other ($\beta = 0.868$, $p < 0.001$, 95% CI $= 0.806$ to 0.926).

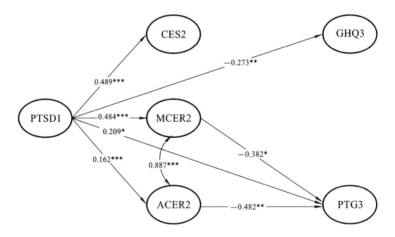

Fig. 4.2　**Model test result for the final model of Study 3 with standardized beta weights added ($n = 757$). Covariates including age, gender, academic stress, initial psychiatric co-morbidity, initial PTG, and PTSD at T3 were controlled for. Only the significant pathways are presented here. $*$ $p < 0.05$, $**$ $p < 0.01$, $***$ $p < 0.001$.**

4.3.3　Mediational Effects

According to the above model results, it was unnecessary to further examine the mediational effect of trauma centrality on the linkages between PTSD and two psychological outcomes. Nor was it necessary to examine the mediational effects of two types of CER on the pathway between PTSD and psychiatric co-morbidity. Instead, the structural model results were implying that adaptive CER and maladaptive CER at T2 might mediate the impact of initial PTSD on posttraumatic growth at T3. Accordingly, mediational analysis revealed that both types of CER at T2 significantly mediated the effect of baseline PTSD on PTG at T3 (adaptive CER: the indirect effect= 0.072, $p<0.05$, 95% CI=0.031 to 0.163; maladaptive CER: the indirect effect=-0.175, $p<0.05$, 95% CI=-0.388 to -0.035).

Considering that the covariates might have explained the variances in psychiatric co-morbidity at T3, leading to the above non-significant relationship between the mediators (i.e. trauma centrality and two types of CER at T2) and psychiatric co-morbidity at T3, we further explored the potential effects that the covariates might have on the results. We re-analyzed the structural model above without controlling for these three covariates (i.e. psychiatric co-morbidity at baseline ($r=0.56$, $p<0.01$), PTSD at T3 ($r=0.63$, $p<0.01$), and academic stress ($r=0.40$, $p<0.01$)) for psychiatric co-morbidity at T3. For the subsequent modified model, there was a good model fit ($\chi^2=1430$, df$=325$, χ^2/df$=4.353$, RMSEA$=0.067$, CFI$= 0.915$, TLI$=0.903$, SRMR$=0.081$). More importantly, in this modified model, adaptive CER and maladaptive CER at T2 were negatively and positively associated with psychiatric co-morbidity at T3, respectively (adaptive CER: $\beta= -0.423$, $p<0.05$, 95% CI=-0.742 to -0.222; maladaptive CER: $\beta=0.525$, $p <0.01$, 95% CI$=0.306$ to 0.921); and both types of CER each mediated the effect of baseline PTSD on psychiatric co-morbidity at T3 (adaptive CER: the indirect effect=-0.067, $p<0.05$, 95% CI=-0.150 to -0.028; maladaptive CER: the indirect effect=0.251, $p<0.05$, 95% CI=0.143 to 0.467).

4.4   Discussion

The current longitudinal study examined the relationship between

PTSD at baseline and negative and positive psychological outcomes at 6-month follow-up (i.e., psychiatric co-morbidity and PTG). It also investigated the mediational effects of trauma centrality, adaptive CER, and maladaptive CER, at 3-month follow-up. Inconsistent with hypothesis 1, after controlling for demographic variables, academic stress, baseline psychiatric co-morbidity, baseline PTG, and PTSD at T3, initial PTSD negatively predicted psychiatric co-morbidity but positively predicted PTG at T3. Partly aligned with hypothesis 2, baseline PTSD was positively associated with trauma centrality at T2 which, however, did not predict the two psychological outcomes at T3 and did not therefore mediate the impact of baseline PTSD onto these two outcomes at T3. Also, partly in line with our third and fourth hypotheses, initial PTSD was positively associated with adaptive CER and maladaptive CER at T2; neither of these two types of CER predicted psychiatric co-morbidity at T3, but both were respectively positively and negatively related to PTG at T3. In addition, both types of CER mediated the pathways between baseline PTSD and PTG at T3 but not those between initial PTSD and psychiatric co-morbidity at T3.

In the current study, 18% and 19% of traumatized adolescents met the DSM-5 screening criteria for probable PTSD at baseline and 6-month follow-up, respectively. These prevalence rates were compatible with the 18% from Study 1 and the 19% from the other study that focused on traumatized adolescents in China (Chen & Chung, 2016). Additional analyses of changes in PTSD diagnostic status over time added to the literature on the trajectory of PTSD symptoms. These findings echoed previous longitudinal studies among hospitalized adolescents exposed to intentional and unintentional injuries (Zatzick et al., 2006) and a community sample of adolescents and young adults (Perkonigg et al., 2005), demonstrating that PTSD symptoms might remit in some individuals but are also likely to persist or exacerbate among others.

Looking at the direct effects of PTSD on psychological outcomes, adolescents with PTSD at baseline experienced greater posttraumatic growth at 6-month follow-up. This finding echoed most studies in the literature (Alisic et al., 2008; Barakat et al., 2006; Hafstad et al., 2010, 2011; Kilmer & Gil-Rivas, 2010; Laufer et al., 2009; Levine et al., 2008; Yu et al., 2010) and supports the assumption that some degrees of posttraumatic distress is a prerequisite for subsequent growth (Nelson, 2011; Tedeschi & Calhoun, 2004). In addition, these traumatized youths also reported less psychiatric comorbidity at 6-month follow-up. Taken together, these direct effects of initial PTSD suggest that our adolescents experienced greater personal growth and psychological well-being at the 6-month follow-up. Following the Janus Face model of PTG (Maercker & Zoellner, 2004), our adolescents may be demonstrating the authentic, self-transcending aspect of growth that facilitates posttraumatic adjustment following a crisis. This self-transforming type of growth is constructive and adaptive. Our adolescents may have facilitated such growth as a coping resource against trauma (Tedeschi et al., 1998; Joseph & Linley, 2004), which in turn may alleviate pain or distress and improve psychological functioning after a crisis (Maercker & Zoellner, 2004).

These adolescents may be resilient individuals and their resilience may have been enhanced by the process of meaning-making as they grow and the Chinese culture (Wang et al., 2020). Meaning-making aims at a better understanding of the trauma and a successful reconciliation of this experience with one's inner structure, which in turn could contribute to recovery. The Chinese collectivist culture in which these adolescents grew up emphasizes the interdependence between family or community members, harmonious relationships with others, and social obligations (Jayawickreme et al., 2013;

Oyserman & Lee, 2008). This could buffer the pathogenic effects of trauma and is therefore often the ideal breeding ground for the development of resilience (Wright et al., 2013). However, this interpretation of resilience in these young people will be revisited later, as the concept of resilience is indeed context-dependent.

Baseline PTSD positively predicted trauma centrality at 3-month follow-up among our adolescent sample, which echoed prior literature among youths (Ionio et al., 2018; Wang et al., 2020). Consistent with the posttraumatic self-hypothesis (Wilson, 2006), PTSD symptoms in this case might have well reflected the basic facets of trauma centrality. This argument was further supported by the strong correlations between the subscales of PTSD and trauma centrality ($r = 0.284$ to 0.386). Somewhat surprisingly, construing trauma as central to their self-concept was not related to the development of subsequent psychiatric co-morbidity or PTG. This aligned with previous evidence of a nonsignificant relation between trauma centrality and PTG among treatment-seeking women (Barton et al., 2013), employees exposed to bombing (Blix et al., 2015), and undergraduates and adults (Taku et al., 2021), but contradicted the findings from other studies (Wang et al., 2020; Schuettler & Boals, 2011; Groleau et al., 2013; Brooks et al., 2017; Chung et al., 2017, 2018).

Moreover, due to the nonsignificant relationship between trauma centrality and the two psychological outcomes in the structural model, trauma centrality could not mediate the impact of initial PTSD onto subsequent psychiatric co-morbidity or PTG. In other words, trauma centrality did not interact with PTSD from past trauma to affect psychological outcomes. Notwithstanding this, as presented above, PTSD from past trauma was directly related to trauma centrality and the two outcomes. Guided by the rationale of the additive model (Chung et al.,

2005), PTSD from past trauma could independently affect the way people view themselves and psychological distress. This unique relationship between PTSD and trauma centrality, in light of the cognitive specificity hypothesis (Beck & Perkins, 2001), might derive from the speculation that PTSD symptoms specifically correspond to the content of thoughts or cognitive processes characterized by trauma centrality. The latter (the content of thoughts or cognitive processes characterized by trauma centrality), however, may not be the cognitive contents peculiar to the development of psychiatric co-morbid symptoms. Thus, no relationship could be established between trauma centrality and psychiatric co-morbidity. Hence, there is no reason to think that PTSD would necessarily impact psychological distress via changes in self-concept.

The additive relationship between PTSD and trauma centrality, as well as between PTSD and psychiatric co-morbidity shed a different light on the trauma centrality hypothesis which postulates that the effects of trauma on mental health outcomes are always channeled through altering victims' personal identity. Similar reasoning could also hold for posttraumatic growth, whereby PTSD from past trauma could contribute to the development of growth and trauma centrality independently. Whilst PTSD symptoms aptly matched the cognitive contents reflected by trauma centrality, these contents of thoughts were not specific to the nurturance of growth. Therefore, the way trauma contributes to positive psychological changes (PTG in this case) is not necessarily channeled through a traumatized schema.

Nevertheless, a different picture emerged when the two types of cognitive emotion regulation (i.e., adaptive CER and maladaptive CER) were taken into account. In terms of adaptive CER, traumatized adolescents resorting to adaptive cognitive emotion regulation at 3-month follow-up reported greater personal growth at 6-month follow-up. This accorded with prior findings that university students with PTSD reported elevated adaptive CER strategies than their counterparts (Slanbekova et al., 2019). It also confirmed the positive relation between adaptive CER strategies and PTG among non-adolescent samples (Hanley et al., 2017; Thomas et al., 2019; Aguirre, 2008; Garnefski et al., 2008; Aflakseir & Manafi, 2018).

Our findings acknowledged the protective role of adaptive CER in facilitating posttraumatic growth out of trauma (Garnefski et al., 2008). Utilizing adaptive CER is about accepting the difficult situation, degrading its severity, appraising it in a more constructive manner, making plans that can best change the situation, and shifting attention to something less threatening. Additional analysis revealed that all these five specific strategies under adaptive CER were positively associated with PTG ($r = 0.127$ to 0.272). Employment of adaptive CER might assist in decentering from the negative view of trauma to its positive aspects, and to the self, and to the world (Koster et al., 2011; Ingram, 1990). This transition may set in motion the regulation of distressing affects and the constructive processing of suppressed memories, so as to enhance understanding of the fearful experience and establish meaningfulness. As such, misbeliefs could be abandoned, unattainable goals be replaced with accessible ones, and existing schema could be revised, giving rise to the phenomenon of posttraumatic growth (Calhoun & Tedeschi, 2006).

Conversely, traumatized adolescents employing more maladaptive CER at 3-month follow-up exhibited less posttraumatic growth at 6-month follow-up. Hereby, the positive prediction of PTSD on maladaptive CER was compatible with previous findings from traumatized adolescents (Amone-P'Olak et al., 2007; Pat-Horenczyk et al., 2014) and adults and emerging adults (Slanbekova et al., 2019; Steel, 2016; Van Loey et al., 2018). Also, our findings confirmed maladaptive cognitive emotion regulation as a risk factor for posttraumatic thriving (Aldao et al., 2010; Garnefski et al., 2001, 2008). Applying maladaptive CER when confronting a crisis could lead victims to blame themselves for the catastrophizing event, exaggerate its terror, and repeatedly reflect on its negative effects (Garnefski et al., 2001). This may narrow victims' attention within the negative context of trauma (Koster et al., 2011; Brewin et al., 1996), alter their perception about the self and others (Janoff-Bulman, 1989, 1992), distort cognitions, and bias the constructive processing of trauma cues (Mathews & MacLeod, 2005). As a result, the resolution of trauma and the assimilation of relevant memories into existing assumptions could be hampered (Joseph & Linley, 2004), undermining the development of personal growth.

However, the structural model showed that utilizing adaptive CER and maladaptive CER at 3-month follow-up did not seem to relate to the severity of psychiatric comorbidity at 6-month follow-up. In other words, neither adaptive CER nor maladaptive CER at 3-month follow-up could mediate the impact of baseline PTSD on subsequent psychiatric comorbidity. This is unexpected, given the well-established positive relation between adaptive CER and psychological well-being and the reverse between maladaptive CER and mental health in previous studies (Amone-P'Olak et al., 2007; d'Acremont & Van der Linden, 2007; Li et al., 2015; Pat-Horenczyk et al., 2013; Garnefski & Kraaij, 2006; Stikkelbroek et al., 2016).

In light of the above discussion, we can now return to the previous claim that these traumatized youth were resilient and would develop greater personal growth and psychological well-being over time. This notion of resilience is indeed context-dependent. For these traumatized adolescents, the degree of resilience in terms of growth or improved psychological well-being depends on the context in which the cognitive emotion coping strategies were used. Some adolescents were resilient in that they seemed to improve their psychological well-being naturally over time, i.e. without relying on specific coping strategies. On the other hand, for some resilient individuals, the extent of their posttraumatic growth depended on whether they used adaptive cognitive emotion coping strategies. These findings may indeed reflect some of the basic tenets of the positive youth hypothesis or "ordinary magic". Resilience is not a rare or special quality. Rather, it springs from the everyday magic of ordinary, normal human resources in their minds, families, and communities (Masten, 2013). For some adolescents in the current study, it seems that their resources have strengthened their overall ability to buffer distress and exhibit psychological well-being despite their trauma. However, the findings also suggest that for other adolescents, certain experiences, in this case, posttraumatic growth, require specific resources such as adaptive cognitive emotion coping strategies.

Some limitations of the present study should be addressed. Firstly, the findings were not based on a random sample. Instead, data collection took place among a convenience sample whose schools were located in the same district of the city and whose classes were selected by their teachers out of convenience. Secondly, these Chinese adolescents' attachment to caregivers (e. g., unresolved attachment) should be taken into account, as a poor relationship with the attachment figure might undermine victims' coping in responding to adversity and affect the development of psychiatric co-morbidity and posttraumatic growth over time. Thirdly, the current study did not control for the potential confounding effect of egocentrism. This is important given that egocentrism is a common phenomenon among adolescents (Elkind, 1967) and might play an important role in their psychological development (Erikson, 1968). Fourthly, the follow-up periods (i.e. six months) for the present study were largely determined by time limit and convenience, not by literature or theories, and may not be long enough to detect the changeability of PTSD symptoms over time. However, we did observe the changes in PTSD diagnosis from baseline to 6-month follow-up among some individuals. Allowing a longer time period, however, may improve future prospective designs to reveal the trajectory of PTSD symptoms over time. Finally, there was an oversight of not controlling academic stress at 6-month follow-up in the present study. Future studies may want to take this into consideration, given the potential effect of academic stress on concurrent psychological well-being.

To conclude, following past trauma, Chinese adolescents can experience psychological distress on one hand and positive changes on the other. Although trauma may redefine adolescents' self-concept and make this event central to their self-understanding, such an alteration did not affect the development of the aforementioned negative and positive outcomes. Moreover, victims' thinking patterns towards trauma did not prove to be a prognostic factor for psychological distress. Instead, this coping strategy influenced the development of positive changes subsequent to crisis. Specifically, thinking positively about the crisis functioned as a protector that promoted its positive effects on personal growth, whereas negative thoughts worked like an inflictor that impaired the emergence of growth.

Chapter 5　Study Four

5.1　Introduction

To recap, the structural model of Study 3 showed that PTSD from past trauma was related to increased posttraumatic growth and reduced psychiatric co-morbidity; whilst PTSD was also associated with strengthened trauma centrality, trauma centrality did not affect the aforesaid psychological outcomes; traumatized adolescents employing adaptive CER displayed greater posttraumatic growth whereas those applying maladaptive CER experienced the reverse; youths' severities of psychiatric co-morbidity were not impacted by their cognitive emotion regulation. These findings imply that the way trauma centrality relates to PTSD is unique and independent of the coping process. Moreover, the coping characterized by cognitive emotion regulation had a significant role to play in the developmental course of PTG following traumatization, which sheds light on the clue that there might exist two types of adolescents (the adaptive copers and the maladaptive copers) when confronting trauma and that these two types of copers may differ in terms of posttraumatic reactions.

5.1.1　PTSD and Unresolved Attachment

Given the important role of attachment relationships on adolescents' traumatic reactions (Liotti, 1992, 1994) and the high prevalence of insecure and unresolved/disorganized attachment among traumatized adolescents and children (Lyons-Ruth et al., 2006; Silva et al., 2000), unresolved attachment, as suggested by the attachment theory (Bowlby, 1980), may provide a valuable approach to understand the posttraumatic responses of these adaptive copers and maladaptive copers following trauma. According to previous work on attachment (Bowlby, 1973, 1980, 1982), humans are born with the tendency to seek proximity to significant others when feeling threatened or distressed. However, although the caregiver may provide love and support to the child, he or she can often behave in a way that is perceived as frightening by the child in daily caregiving. The child will then on one hand want to approach the caregiver, but at the same time be afraid to do so, which gradually leads to the formation of negative schematic representations of the self (as being unlovable) and of significant others (as being indifferent, unavailable, and unresponsive, or even being cruel or abusive) (Bowlby, 1973). In extreme cases, these negative internal working models could lead to disorganized or unresolved representations (Bowlby, 1982; Main & Hesse, 1990; Simpson & Rholes, 2002), whereby victims' attachment behaviors are disorganized, and display the incompatible approach-avoidant pattern in times of need or distress. These schematic representations can be conceptualized as a form of unresolved attachment that is stored in victims' autobiographical memory systems and will be automatically activated to shape their interactions with the same attachment figure or other partners in future times of stress (e.g., being exposed to trauma) (Horowitz, 1982; Mikulincer et al., 2002; Bowlby, 1973).

Unresolved attachment could interweave with PTSD symptoms among traumatized individuals. As illustrated earlier, trauma can activate the victim's system of unresolved attachment. This is an attachment system that lacks inner models of comfort-providing figures and external sources of support to protect oneself from the pathogenic effects of trauma. As a result, strong negative feelings of rejection, loneliness and helplessness might be induced, that could heighten posttraumatic suffering. Also, given that unresolved individuals' affect regulation capacities tend to be impaired and underdeveloped (Brier, 2002), to avoid severe disruption to self-concept, they may rely on the less effective strategies of hyperactivating and deactivating to cope with the overwhelming trauma (Mikulincer et al., 2015). The former (hyperactivating) promotes the reactivation of and rumination over trauma memories, but the latter (deactivating) drives the denial of traumatic distress and the avoidance of potential reminders. Together, these maladaptive emotion regulation skills could contribute to or intensify intrusive and avoidance reactions respectively, thus preventing the resolution of trauma and predisposing unresolved victims to long-term struggles with PTSD (Mikulincer et al., 2015). Furthermore, prolonged and pervasive PTSD could also intensify victims' sense of unresolved attachment. In this case, the frequent unwanted intrusive memories, dreams, or flashbacks function like constant reminders of the traumatic experience, which could reinforce victims' beliefs about the untrustworthiness of others and the danger of the world, continue to shatter their assumptions about self-capabilities, and exacerbate the sense of helplessness and vulnerability. These negative views about oneself and others and the concomitant feelings of helplessness and vulnerability would only amplify their awareness of the presence of their internal unresolved attachment experiences (Mikulincer et al., 2015).

Despite the existing research on the relationship between PTSD and unresolved attachment in adults (Stovall-McClough & Cloitre, 2006; Nye et al., 2008; Harari et al., 2009; Riggs et al., 2007; Turton et al., 2004) and children (MacDonald et al., 2008), only one study has so far investigated this among adolescents (Joubert et al., 2012). Specifically, the authors focused on a group of adolescent survivors of child abuse and revealed a positive relation between unresolved attachment and trauma symptoms (Joubert et al., 2012). Clearly, more research is needed to explore this link among adolescents, especially those in China.

5.1.2   Unresolved Attachment and Psychiatric Co-morbidity

Unresolved attachment can also be a contributor to psychiatric co-morbid symptoms. Guided by attachment theory (Bowlby, 1982), unresolved attachment reflects inadequate love and protection from significant others during times of distress or stress, which does not provide a secure base from which victims can learn to handle their painful internal states through trial and error (Briere, 1996). As such, the establishment of a progressively more mature repertoire of affect modulation may be impaired, resulting in insufficient capacities for affect tolerance and underdeveloped capabilities for emotion regulation (Bowlby, 1980; Briere, 1996, 2002). This undermined affect modulation or tolerance is, however, incapable of adequately managing the negative affect arousals from trauma. Although these individuals might resort to the aforementioned anxious hyperactivation and avoidance deactivation to assist continuous psychological functioning, such strategies, as elucidated earlier, were maladaptive in nature and could disrupt the support-seeking and relational interdependence required by successful resolution of distress (Mikulincer & Shaver, 2003). As such, unresolved attachment could interfere with affect modulation to deteriorate psychological functioning, which in turn might place unresolved victims at a heightened risk for depression and anxiety during the posttraumatic period (Mikulincer et al., 2015). Indeed, preliminary evidence of adolescents with unresolved attachment also reporting escalated depressive symptoms has emerged (van Hoof et al., 2015; Ivarsson et al., 2010). However, given the paucity of research on the association between unresolved attachment and psychological distress among youths, it is important to revisit this investigation with other adolescent samples.

5.1.3 Unresolved Attachment and Posttraumatic Growth

Theoretically speaking, unresolved attachment can also be associated with posttraumatic growth. Subsequent to a crisis, unresolved individuals may not have supportive others to turn to for disclosing about their traumatic experience. As a result, they have never incorporated into their schema the positive and constructive experiences of supportive others. However, this kind of constructive schema is needed for the development of posttraumatic growth (Tedeschi & Calhoun, 2004). Besides, others' comfort and support during disclosure could strengthen the intimacy between the victim and the listener, relieve victims' emotional distress, enhance tolerance for negative affects, and facilitate emotional equanimity (Tedeschi & Calhoun, 2004; Calhoun & Tedeschi, 2006). By contrast, a lack of supportive others in the cases of unresolved attachment, along with the pre-existing affect modulation impairment, might result in failures in the above emotion regulation (Mikulincer & Shaver, 2007), which in turn could hamper subsequent cognitive readjusting of trauma materials and the ascription of meaning (Tedeschi & Calhoun, 2004; Calhoun & Tedeschi, 2006; Joubert et al., 2012), thereby undermining the experience of posttraumatic growth. Nevertheless, the relationship between unresolved attachment and posttraumatic growth has not been explored in the literature.

5.1.4 Egocentrism and Psychological Outcomes

Egocentrism, a salient phenomenon among adolescents, might

potentially influence the aforementioned negative and positive psychological outcomes. Egocentrism reflects distorted cognitions (Elkind, 1985) and is defined by adolescents seeing the self as being unique and invulnerable across occasions (the personal fable), perceiving others closely watching, evaluating, criticizing, and admiring them as much as they do themselves (the imaginary audience), and centering attention, thoughts, beliefs, and feelings inward to the self as opposed to outward, i.e., to other people or the external (general self-focuses) (Elkind, 1967). Under the function of these three components, egocentrism may contribute to the etiology of general psychological distress in the aftermath of trauma (Elkind, 1985). Specifically, by personal fable, traumatized victims might deny their vulnerability (e.g., loss and posttraumatic stress symptoms) during the presence of trauma, maintain their fake uniqueness and powerfulness in a negative way, and refuse social support and medical assistance. In terms of the imaginary audience, adolescents might fantasize about this audience, preoccupy themselves with the potential regard of these people, and even come to share the negative comments that they imagine their audience makes about them. The aforementioned denial of loss/symptoms and rejection of care disallow negative affects to be emotionally processed and the imagined negative evaluations from others might induce additional destructive feelings, all of which could accumulate emotional distress and aggravate psychological suffering. Moreover, the general self-focus component of egocentrism is characterized by excessive attention being continuously directed towards the self and the inner world but a disregard for external demands. As a result, this disruption in attention deployment could exacerbate psychopathological symptoms such as blaming oneself and being engulfed in negative affects, thoughts, and beliefs associated with one's traumatic experience (Ingram, 1990). Not surprisingly, egocentric adolescents reported escalated depression and anxiety symptoms (Baron, 1986; Garber et al., 1993).

Also, egocentrism could exert some influence on the formation of posttraumatic growth. The three components of egocentrism, as illustrated above, were associated with the accumulation of emotional distress which, if beyond tolerance, was likely to hamper the subsequent cognitive readjusting processes associated with the development of PTG (Tedeschi & Calhoun, 2004). Additionally, victims' denial and avoidance of trauma cues and their illusory invulnerability (derived from personal fable) might discourage constructive processing of unresolved information and support seeking, both of which, however, are important elements in PTG theories to facilitate posttraumatic growth (Tedeschi & Calhoun, 2004; Calhoun & Tedeschi, 2006). Finally, the general self-focus component tends to hinder attention on event-relevant tasks such as the processing of trauma or on the positive aspects of the event (Ingram, 1990; Koster et al., 2011). As a result, the issues pertaining to trauma are not resolved, and potential benefits or growth are not gained (Calhoun & Tedeschi, 2006).

5.1.5 Aims and Hypotheses

What was postulated above set the theoretical base for the current study. By focusing on a group of Chinese adolescents with past trauma, the current study intended to explore whether PTSD from past trauma could co-exist with cognitive emotion regulation and unresolved attachment to influence psychological outcomes characterized by psychiatric co-morbidity and posttraumatic growth. Latent Profile Analysis (LPA), a person-centered approach, was the appropriate method for this purpose. LPA, based on the response patterns of PTSD, cognitive emotion regulation, and unresolved attachment, can uncover subgroups of adolescents who share similarities in response patterns. For instance, one subgroup of adolescents with a certain level of PTSD symptoms might at the same time display certain levels of difficulties in attachment, adopting certain styles of cognitive emotion regulation (e.g., more adaptive CER and less maladaptive CER, or the reverse, or other styles). Whilst similar response patterns could be observed within each subgroup, different patterns would be observed between subgroups. In other words, homogeneity can be found between adolescents within each subgroup, and heterogeneity between individuals in different subgroups (Lubke & Muthen, 2007). Following LPA, subsequent analysis can explore to what extent these subgroups differ in psychological outcomes. That is, latent profile analysis could reveal how different patterns or clusters of symptoms would affect mental health outcomes, which is different from regression analysis. The latter only tells us which variable has the most salient effect on outcomes, which is not the aim of the current study. Instead, the study aimed to investigate how concurrent experiences, characterized by past trauma, past attachment difficulties with significant others, and intrinsic emotion regulation strategies, cohered to influence psychological outcomes. This might advance our understanding about the results from Study 3. Additionally, information of the suffering and characteristics of a certain subgroup could facilitate tailored treatment for that particular group of victims and improve treatment efficiency when applied to group therapy. To the best of our knowledge, no studies have thus far used LPA to display different patterns of PTSD, unresolved attachment, and cognitive emotion regulation among adolescents, and how these patterns would influence negative and positive psychological outcomes measured as psychiatric co-morbidity and posttraumatic growth.

Similar to Study 3, adolescents' demographic information and academic stress needed to be controlled for in the current study. We additionally took into account egocentrism, which is an endemic cognitive symptom among adolescents (Elkind, 1967). As illustrated earlier, the cognitive distortions incurred by egocentrism could interfere with emotion regulation and bias the cognitive readjusting of traumatic information, in turn affecting posttraumatic adaptation outcomes like psychiatric co-morbidity (Elkind, 1985; Baron, 1986; Garber et al., 1993) and posttraumatic growth (Tedeschi & Calhoun, 2004). Hence, after controlling for demographic variables and the levels of academic stress and egocentrism, we hypothesized as follows:

(1) There would be distinct subgroups of adolescents with different profiles of co-occurring PTSD, CER, and unresolved attachment;

(2) These distinct subgroups would differ in the psychological outcomes of posttraumatic growth and co-morbid psychiatric symptoms.

5.2 Methods

5.2.1 Participants and Procedure

Data collection for the present study was based on a convenience sample recruited from two secondary schools (one junior high school and one senior high school) in China. After explaining the purpose and procedures of the study to the principals of these two schools and obtaining permission (written consent), the researcher visited the two psychology teachers and ten course teachers at these schools. These twelve teachers assisted the researcher in identifying eligible adolescents from the classes they teach. The inclusion criteria were 1) of Chinese ethnicity, and 2) having enrolled at the participating schools, as confirmed by the school registers. Participants who met the criteria were then met in their respective classrooms during the course times of the twelve teachers, debriefed about the study, given a battery of self-report questionnaires (see "Measures") to complete in class, and ensured the anonymity of their participation and the confidentiality of their submitted information. They were also reminded of their right to withdraw from the study whenever they wanted. Students provided consent before participating. After data collection, students were thanked, and similar to the previous two studies, their psychology teachers at school were invited to provide counselling services to participants in need. All of the questionnaires were distributed in Chinese following the same back-translation procedure as illustrated in Study 1. Ethical approval was obtained from the Survey and Behavioral Research Ethics Committee at the Chinese University of Hong Kong.

Missing data of more than 20% on a key variable was considered unacceptable (Parent, 2013), therefore, sixty-six questionnaires were excluded. Of the 1057 valid assessments, 108 did not indicate any past trauma; therefore, they were also excluded. A final sample of nine hundred and forty-nine ($n = 949$; male $= 487$, female $= 462$) eligible participants was included for the present study. Of them, 13%, 27%, and 10% were the first, second, and third graders in junior middle school, respectively; and 21%, 18%, and 11% were the first, second, and third graders in senior high school, respectively. On average, our participants were 15 years old ($\mu_{age} = 14.63$, $S = 1.66$, range $= 12$ to 19), of Chinese origin, and did not receive any special needs education.

5. 2. 2   Measures

Demographic information, Posttraumatic stress disorder, Psychiatric co-morbidity, Posttraumatic growth, and Academic stress

For the measurement of these constructs, the same instruments as described in Study 2 were adopted in Study 4. Based on the current sample, the Cronbach's alpha for the total score of PTSD was 0.94; for the total score of psychiatric co-morbidity was 0.95; for the total score of PTG was 0.94; and for the total score of academic stress was 0.90. Cognitive emotion regulation was evaluated using the same instrument as illustrated in Study 3. Based on the current sample, the Cronbach's alpha for CER total score, adaptive CER subscale, and maladaptive CER subscale were 0.89, 0.86, and 0.82, respectively.

Egocentrism

The Adolescent Egocentrism-Sociocentrism Scale (AES; Enright et al., 1980) is a 45-item measure of egocentrism, sociocentrism, and nonsocial focus among adolescents. In the current study, only the egocentrism dimension is of interest. It includes 15 items and consists of three components: the personal fable (e.g., accepting the fact that others don't know what it's like being me), the imaginary audience (when walking in late to a group meeting, trying not to distract everyone's attention), and general self-focuses (becoming real good at being able to think through my own thoughts). Each component is assessed by 5 items. Adolescents read each item and decide to what extent the statement is important to him/her in a 5-point Likert response format ranging from 1 (what the statement implies is of no importance to me) to 5 (what the statement concerns is of great importance to me). A total score per component is acquired by adding up the scores of all items in that component. This scale also yields a total score for egocentrism (a sum of all the 15 items' scores, range = 15-75), which indicates the overall degree of being egocentric. Previous studies among adolescents in the US demonstrated adequate internal consistency and good reliabilities with a Cronbach's alpha for the egocentrism subscale being 0.78 (Enright et al., 1979), 0.83 (Enright et al., 1980), and 0.88 (Frankenberger,

2004), respectively. Based on the current sample, the Cronbach's alpha for the total score of egocentrism was 0.83.

Unresolved attachment

The Adolescent Unresolved Attachment Questionnaire (AUAQ; West et al., 2000) first asks adolescents to identify a primary attachment figure who is mainly responsible for raising them in their day-to-day lives. This person can be their father, mother, grandfather, grandmother, or someone else. Following that, the scale presents 10 items to evaluate adolescents' perception of attachment difficulties with this primary attachment figure as well as related negative emotional responses to such failure. This self-report instrument comprises three subscales, i.e., failed protection (4 items, e.g., when I'm upset, I am sure that my parent will be there to listen to me), anger/dysregulation (3 items, e.g., I think it is unfair to always have to handle problems by myself), and fear (3 items, e.g., I'm afraid that I will lose my parent's love). Adolescents read each statement and answer to what extent they agree with the statement on a 5-point Likert scale ranging from 1 (strongly disagree) to 5 (strongly agree). A total score for each subscale is obtained by summing up all the items under that subscale. This scale has shown acceptable validity and reliability among adolescents with the Cronbach's alpha for the three subscales being 0.71 (failed protection), 0.73 (anger/dysregulation), and 0.66 (fear), respectively (West et al., 2000). Based on the current sample, the Cronbach's alpha for the total score of unresolved attachment was 0.82.

5.2.3 **Statistical Analysis**

Descriptive statistics and multivariate analyses of variance (MANOVA) were conducted in SPSS 25. Latent Profile Analysis, a person-centered approach, was also carried out in Mplus 7.4 to explore unobservable subgroups of adolescents organized by symptom presentation patterns of co-occurring PTSD, cognitive emotion regulation, and unresolved attachment. In other words, LPA classifies traumatized adolescents into several homogeneous subgroups based on their similarities in symptom severity of PTSD, cognitive emotion regulation, and unresolved attachment. For the facilitation of model convergence and the ease of interpreting LPA results (Au et al., 2013), subscales of PTSD (intrusion, avoidance, negative alterations in cognition and mood, and alterations in arousal and reactivity), cognitive emotion regulation (adaptive CER and maladaptive CER), and the total score of unresolved attachment were employed to create profile patterns in LPA. To enhance the interpretability of latent profile solutions, the scores of PTSD subscales, CER subscales, and unresolved attachment total were standardized prior to being used for model estimation. The robust maximum likelihood estimator (MLE) was preferred as the appropriate fit function.

The following fit indices were adopted for model comparisons: a lower Akaike Information Criterion (AIC), a lower Bayesian Information Criterion (BIC), a lower sample-size adjusted Bayesian Information Criterion (aBIC) value, a significant Bootstrap likelihood ratio test (BLRT, $p < 0.05$), a significant Lo-Mendell-Rubin adjusted likelihood ratio test (LMR-A, $p < 0.05$) which signifies that the k classes model is superior to the $k-1$ classes model, and a higher entropy which indicates that the corresponding profile solution is accurate and acceptable (Nylund et al., 2007). We also took into account parsimony, class quality, and substantive significance when identifying the optimal profile pattern. For the current study, one to six models were generated to facilitate comparison.

The most likely class membership suggested by the optimal solution was then imported into SPSS 25 as an independent variable for overall psychiatric co-morbidity (the GHQ-28 total score) and overall posttraumatic growth (the PTGI total score). With demographic variables, levels of academic stress, and egocentrism adjusted, multivariate analyses of variance (MANOVA) examined differences in overall psychiatric co-morbidity and posttraumatic growth across profiles. Similar to Study 1, the effect sizes were estimated using partial eta-squared statistics and evaluated according to Cohen's suggestion (1988), with 0. 010-0. 058 being small, 0. 059-0. 137 being medium, and 0. 138 and above being large.

5.3　Results

5.3.1　Descriptive Statistics and Correlation

Using the PCL-5, 25% of students reported one trauma and 75% experienced multiple traumas. The most frequently reported event was the sudden death of someone close (68%), followed by transportation accident (60%), life-threatening illness (36%), and physical assault (30%). The most bothering event happened on average 3. 90 ($S = 3. 25$) years ago. According to the DSM-5 screening criteria, 23%, 52%, and 25% of our participants were classified into the probable PTSD, mild-moderate PTSD, and no PTSD group, respectively.

Pearson's correlational analysis revealed that being female and perceiving greater academic stress were related to higher levels of co-morbid psychiatric symptoms (gender (0 = male, 1 = female): $r = 0. 18, p < 0. 01$; academic stress: $r = 0. 52, p < 0. 01$) and lower levels of PTG (gender: $r = -0. 07, p < 0. 05$; academic stress: $r = -0. 16, p < 0. 01$). Older students would experience more severe co-morbid psychiatric symptoms ($r = 0. 15, p < 0. 01$) but not greater PTG ($r = 0. 03, p > 0. 05$). Being more egocentric was not related to psychiatric symptoms ($r = 0. 06, p > 0. 05$) but was associated with more growth ($r = 0. 28, p < 0. 01$). Hence, in addition to academic stress and ecocentrism, age and gender would also be controlled for as covariates in subsequent analyses.

5.3.2　Multivariate Test between Diagnostic Groups

MANOVA revealed significant differences between these three groups in adaptive and maladaptive CER, unresolved attachment, co-morbid psychiatric symptoms, and PTG. The probable PTSD group reported significantly higher levels of adaptive CER, maladaptive CER, unresolved attachment, and co-morbid psychiatric symptoms, but lower levels of PTG than the mild-moderate PTSD (adaptive CER: 95% CI = 0.24 to 3.21; maladaptive CER: 95% CI = 6.16 to 8.01; attachment: 95% CI = 3.07 to 5.26; psychiatric symptoms: 95% CI = 15.32 to 19.45; PTG: 95% CI = −12.48 to −5.44) and the no PTSD group (adaptive CER: 95% CI = 3.01 to 6.44; maladaptive CER: 95% CI = 9.80 to 11.93; attachment: 95% CI = 6.41 to 8.94; psychiatric symptoms: 95% CI = 21.46 to 26.24; PTG: 95% CI = −13.55 to −5.41) (see Table 5.1).

Table 5.1　Means and standard deviations of adaptive CER, maladaptive CER, unresolved attachment, psychiatric co-morbidity, and PTG between three diagnostic groups (n = 949).

	Probable PTSD μ (S)	Mild-moderate PTSD μ (S)	No PTSD μ (S)	F	Post hoc analyses $p < 0.05$	Partial η^2
Adaptive CER	30.38 (7.78)	28.66 (9.09)	25.65 (11.02)	15.31***	No<Mild-moderate <Probable	0.031
Maladaptive CER	24.27 (6.09)	17.19 (5.86)	13.40 (5.47)	206.44***	No<Mild-moderate <Probable	0.304
UA	26.23 (7.23)	22.07 (7.06)	18.56 (6.19)	70.79***	No<Mild-moderate <Probable	0.130

Continue

	Probable PTSD μ (S)	Mild-moderate PTSD μ (S)	No PTSD μ (S)	F	Post hoc analyses $p<0.05$	Partial η^2
Co-morbid psychiatric symptoms	67.05 (14.54)	49.67 (13.20)	43.21 (10.87)	209.99***	No<Mild-moderate <Probable	0.307
PTG	48.14 (20.26)	57.11 (21.63)	57.62 (24.79)	14.44***	Probable <Mild-moderate=No	0.030

Note: *** $p < 0.001$. See List of Abbreviations for variable names.

5.3.3   Latent Profile Models

The model-fitting results of six LPA models using the subscales of PTSD and CER and the total score of disorganized attachment were presented in Table 5.2. The 1-class model, with no entropy, no LMR-A, and no BLRT values, was apparently inadvisable. The 2,3, and 4-class models were superior to the 5 and 6-class solutions as the 2,3, and 4-class models produced significant and marginally significant LMR-A values. Further comparisons between the 2,3, and 4-class models favored the 4-class solution given its lower AIC, BIC, and aBIC values, higher class quality, greater substantive significance, and high entropy. Hence, the 4-class model was identified as the optimal solution.

Table 5.2   Fit indices for LPA models using subscale scores of PTSD and cognitive emotion regulation and the total score of unresolved attachment ($n=949$).

Model	AIC	BIC	aBIC	Entropy	LMR-A	BLRT
1-class	19 136.86	19 204.84	19 160.38	—	—	—
2-class	16 759.17	16 865.99	16 796.12	0.91	<0.001	<0.001

Continue

Model	AIC	BIC	aBIC	Entropy	LMR-A	BLRT
3-class	16 119.92	16 265.59	16 170.31	0.89	<0.001	<0.001
4-class	**15 933.20**	**16 117.70**	**15 997.02**	**0.80**	**0.05**	**<0.001**
5-class	15 775.10	15 998.45	15 852.36	0.80	0.36	<0.001
6-class	15 641.18	15 903.37	15 731.87	0.81	0.20	<0.001

Note: The words and numbers in bold indicate the optimal model. AIC= Akaike Information Criterion;

BIC= Bayesian Information Criterion; aBIC = adjusted Bayesian Information Criterion; LMR-A = Lo-

Mendell-Rubin adjusted likelihood ratio test; BLRT: Bootstrap likelihood ratio test.

5.3.4 The Optimal Model

The 4-class model is depicted in Fig. 5.1 and presents low trauma group (Class 1, $n = 290, 30\%$), adaptive coping group (Class 2, $n = 252, 27\%$), moderate trauma group (Class 3, $n = 283, 30\%$), and high trauma group (Class 4, $n = 124, 13\%$).

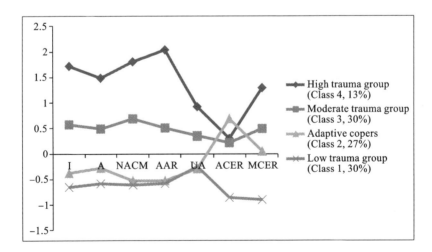

Fig. 5.1   **The 4-class model for Study 4 ($n = 949$) using standardized subscale scores of PTSD and cognitive emotion regulation and standardized total score of unresolved attachment.**

With demographics (i.e., gender and age) and levels of academic stress

and egocentrism adjusted for, MANOVA then examined whether the four distinct subgroups would differ in outcomes of PTG and co-morbid psychiatric symptoms (see Table 5.3). Results indicated that Class 4 suffered greater severities of co-morbid psychiatric symptoms than did Class 3 (95% CI=10.30 to 14.94), Class 2 (95% CI=21.24 to 26.14), and Class 1 (95% CI = 21.68 to 26.61). Class 3 demonstrated higher levels of co-morbid psychiatric symptoms than Class 2 (95% CI=9.20 to 12.94) and Class 1 (95% CI=9.68 to 13.37), whereas these latter two classes did not differ in psychiatric symptom severity (95% CI = −1.39 to 2.30). Conversely, with respect to posttraumatic growth, Class 4 students reported significantly lower levels than Class 3 (95% CI=−11.12 to −2.52), Class 2 (95% CI=−24.43 to −15.34), and Class 1 individuals (95% CI=−9.45 to −0.31). Class 3 experienced comparable levels of PTG with Class 1 (95% CI=−1.49 to 5.37), and these two classes displayed lower levels of PTG than Class 2 (Class 3 vs. Class 2: 95% CI=−16.53 to −9.60; Class 1 vs. Class 2: 95% CI=−18.42 to −11.59).

Table 5.3   Results of MANOVA using class membership as the independent variable, and co-morbid psychiatric symptoms and PTG as dependent variables ($n=949$).

	Class 1 μ (S)	Class 2 μ (S)	Class 3 μ (S)	Class 4 μ (S)	Sample μ (S)	F	Post hoc analyses $p<0.05$	Partial η^2
Co-morbid psychiatric symptoms	43.43 (10.47)	45.09 (11.13)	58.12 (12.47)	72.99 (14.46)	52.11 (15.61)	159.63***	1=2<3<4	0.34
PTG	51.12 (23.50)	67.40 (18.41)	52.72 (21.33)	45.20 (19.96)	55.15 (22.47)	37.10***	4<3=1<2	0.11

Note: *** $p<0.001$; PTG = posttraumatic growth; Class 1=low trauma group; Class 2 = adaptive coping group; Class 3=moderate trauma group; Class 4=high trauma group.

5.4　Discussion

Based on a group of Chinese adolescents with past trauma, the present study examined two hypotheses: 1) there would be distinct subgroups of adolescents with different profiles of co-occurring PTSD, CER, and unresolved attachment; and 2) these distinct subgroups would differ in terms of posttraumatic growth and co-morbid psychiatric symptoms. Consistent with the first hypothesis, four non-parallel profiles of adolescents were identified: the low trauma group (Class 1), the adaptive coping group (Class 2), the moderate trauma group (Class 3), and the high trauma group (Class 4). Consistent with the second hypothesis, these four distinct classes differed in terms of PTG and co-morbid psychiatric symptoms. Adolescents in the high trauma group had more severe co-morbid psychiatric symptoms and lower levels of PTG than individuals in the other three groups.

The fact that adolescents in Class 4 (high trauma group) reported significantly more severe co-morbid psychiatric symptoms than those in Class 3 (moderate trauma group) might be due to the dose-response hypothesis (Dohrenwend & Dohrenwend, 1974). This hypothesis states that the magnitude of trauma and dysfunctional defenses may impact the severity of the individual's (in this case, the traumatized adolescent's) psychological distress, i.e., the higher the magnitude, the worse the well-being (Johnson & Thompson, 2008). Additional analysis revealed a significantly higher magnitude of PTSD symptoms (Class 4 vs. Class 3: intrusion, 14. 67 vs. 8. 90, $p<0.001$; avoidance, 6. 00 vs. 3. 46, $p<0.001$; NACM, 18. 49 vs. 11. 32, $p<0.001$; AAR, 16. 05 vs. 7. 63, $p<0.001$), unresolved attachment (Class 4 vs. Class 3: 28. 72 vs. 24. 33, $p<0.001$), and maladaptive CER (Class 4 vs. Class 3: 26. 54 vs. 20. 78, $p<0.001$) among students in the high trauma group than those in the moderate trauma group, and comparable adaptive CER (Class 4 vs. Class 3; 31. 09 vs. 29. 82, $p > 0.05$) in both groups. This result echoed past findings of the negative impacts of PTSD, unresolved attachment, and maladaptive CER on co-morbid psychiatric symptoms among diverse traumatized adolescents (Amone-P'Olak et al., 2007; Garnefski & Kraaij, 2006; Ivarsson et al., 2010; van Hoof et al., 2015).

Conversely, adolescents in Class 4 (high trauma group) reported significantly lower levels of PTG than adolescents in Class 3 (moderate trauma group). This may confirm earlier PTG literature indicating that too much distress (e.g., high levels of trauma) is unfavorable for the development and maintenance of posttraumatic growth, whereas moderate levels of distress are (Calhoun & Tedeschi, 2006). This makes sense, as high levels of distress would exceed an individual's capacity for tolerance and regulation. To prevent exhaustion, traumatized adolescents might develop emotional numbness and cognitive and behavioral avoidance to escape trauma cues and their associated negative affects, rather than constructively process these cues and emotions. This may hinder understanding of the trauma and discourage benefit finding from this fearful experience, thereby hindering the development of posttraumatic growth (Calhoun & Tedeschi, 2006). However, with moderate distress, the negative emotional arousal can be relatively easier to be reduced and tolerated. This reduction in distress paves the way for and initiates subsequent cognitive processing of trauma cues, which in turn may contribute to the accumulation of PTG (Cann et al., 2010).

As shown above, adolescents in the high trauma group also reported higher levels of unresolved attachment and maladaptive CER than adolescents in the moderate trauma group. The former (unresolved attachment) was associated with impaired capacities of affect modulation and tolerance (Bowlby, 1980) and inadequate or even absent support from significant others (Bowlby, 1980; Mikulincer et al., 2002), both of which, however, would prevent the restoration of emotional balance and hinder the cognitive processing of suppressed memories. The latter (maladaptive CER) was prone to interfere with the reduction of distress and distort the processing of trauma material (Aldao et al., 2010; Garnefski et al., 2008). Together, these two (unresolved attachment and maladaptive CER) might prevent the revision of existing schemas and the production of meaning, thus reducing the likelihood of posttraumatic growth (Tedeschi & Calhoun, 2004). This finding aligns with previous longitudinal research that found maladaptive CER in traumatized adolescents at 3 months negatively predicted PTG at 6 months (Wang, Chung, Liu, et al., 2022). Moreover, our findings add to the literature that unresolved attachment may negatively influence posttraumatic growth and positively influence co-morbid psychiatric symptoms.

Our finding that adolescents in Class 2 (adaptive coping group) and Class 1 (low trauma group) suffered from co-morbid psychiatric symptoms to a lesser extent might be due to the low severity of trauma and attachment crisis in both groups. The lower the level of distress, the fewer the mental health problems (Dohrenwend & Dohrenwend, 1974; Johnson & Thompson, 2008). Furthermore, when looking at the profiles of these two classes, we find that whilst the adaptive coping group showed slightly more frequent intrusions and avoidance (Class 2 vs. Class 1: intrusion, 4.34 vs. 2.73, $p <$ 0.001; avoidance, 1.58 vs. 0.76, $p < 0.001$; NACM, 3.32 vs. 2.88, $p > 0.$ 05; AAR, 1.87 vs. 1.78, $p > 0.05$; unresolved attachment, 19.42 vs. 19.64, $p >$ 0.05), both classes suffered from comparable levels of co-morbid psychiatric distress. This could be related to the fact that the adaptive coping group applied higher levels of adaptive CER (Class 2 vs. Class 1: 35.58 vs. 19.33,

$p<0.001$), as adaptive CER reflects efficient coping with the pathogenic effects of trauma (Garnefski et al., 2008), which in turn could alleviate the distress caused by the slightly higher levels of intrusion and avoidance, thus improving psychological well-being to almost the same extent as the low trauma group. This finding is consistent with previous research showing that adaptive cognitive emotion regulation is an important protective factor for adolescent mental health (Amone-P'Olak et al., 2007; Garnefski & Kraaij, 2006; Li et al., 2015).

Despite similar levels of co-morbid psychiatric symptoms, the adaptive coping group and the low trauma group experienced different levels of posttraumatic growth. The profiles of these two groups indicated a higher representation of intrusion and avoidance symptoms in the adaptive copers, who, however, used more adaptive CER strategies and consequently experienced greater posttraumatic growth. These findings suggest that the adaptive copers may be resilient individuals (Masten, 2014). They tended to perceive their traumatic experiences and attachment difficulties as less severe, and they may have a natural tendency to cope with the above crises using more adaptive strategies.

This speculation was confirmed by our results from additional analyses. While adaptive CER was positively correlated with all five subscales of PTG for each of the two classes, the strengths of these correlations were stronger in the adaptive coping group ($r=0.29$ to 0.41, $p<0.05$) than in the low trauma group ($r=0.12$ to 0.26, $p<0.05$). These stronger correlation coefficients may suggest some intrinsic motivation behind the phenomenon of posttraumatic growth that drives adaptive copers to deal with trauma in more constructive ways, for example, by down-regulating trauma-related negative affect to promote subsequent cognitive processing/readjustment of suppressed trauma memories (Tedeschi & Calhoun, 2004). The latter (cognitive readjustment) may be somewhat related to the process of deliberate rumination, which aims to make sense of trauma (Cann et al., 2010; Joseph & Linley, 2004). A better understanding about the trauma could in turn drive the revision of the existing schema and facilitate the meaning-making associated with the improvement of PTG (Tedeschi & Calhoun, 2004).

In contrast, the low trauma group had the lowest scores for PTSD and unresolved attachment representations and were least likely to use adaptive and maladaptive CER strategies. Therefore, the low trauma group might not feel the need to rely heavily on cognitive emotion regulation due to their low trauma and limited attachment problems. In other words, the individuals in the low trauma group may not have been challenged or tested by high levels of negative experiences (i.e., trauma and unresolved attachment issues). This group could almost be treated as a control group for the present study.

Several limitations of the current study should be acknowledged. Firstly, our study was based on a convenience sample recruited from two secondary schools in the same district. Therefore, the generalizability of the findings to other adolescents and clinical samples might be questioned. Secondly, the current study is a cross-sectional study, which is unable to detect profile changes over time due to the lack of temporal precedence (Cole & Maxwell, 2003). Future studies with a longitudinal design could better address this. Thirdly, unresolved attachment was assessed using self-report instruments rather than the traditional Adult Attachment Interview (AAI) by mental health professionals, which may have introduced some bias. However, as the AAI is very demanding in terms of the expertise and time required for discourse analysis, the AUAQ might be more appropriate for large-scale studies aimed only at capturing the relational phenomena of unresolved attachment (West et al., 2000).

To conclude, Chinese adolescents may experience both emotional distress and personal growth following catastrophic events. The extent of these psychological responses could be influenced by the interactions between the adolescents' past trauma experiences, adaptive and maladaptive coping, and attachment difficulties. In other words, the adolescents' past traumatic memories, their past experiences with attachment figures, and how they cope could influence psychological problems and growth. These past experiences are often beyond the individual's control, while coping tends to reflect conscious behaviors or activities that are usually within the adolescent's control. Future studies could further explore the role of loss of control and being in control on mental health after trauma.

Chapter 6 General Discussion

This chapter presents an overall discussion on the main findings of the four consecutive studies. In general, our results are aligned with the theoretical frameworks of the PTG model and the self-trauma model and have extended these two models by incorporating the impacts of trauma centrality, cognitive emotion regulation, and unresolved attachment. Implications of the findings and directions for future research are also discussed.

6.1 Recap Main Findings of the Four Studies

Focusing on Chinese adolescents with a history of traumatic exposure, the present thesis has combined retrospective and prospective designs to investigate the relationship between PTSD from past trauma, trauma centrality, cognitive emotion regulation, unresolved attachment, and psychological outcomes (i.e., psychiatric co-morbidity and posttraumatic growth). Several main findings are worth noting.

First, the four studies revealed that around 54%-66% of adolescents were exposed to at least one type of trauma in the past, which is compatible with prior findings (46%-94%) among other traumatized Chinese youths (Wang & Chung, 2020; Chen & Chung, 2016; Wang et al., 2017; Wang et al., 2021; Yu et al., 2020; Xiao et al., 2021; Chan, 2013). These figures suggested that trauma exposure was statistically normative within the adolescent population. Following trauma, the prevalence rates for probable

PTSD varied between 17% and 20% across the four studies, and these were similar to previous rates of 19% (Chung & Chen, 2017) and 21% (Chen & Chung, 2016) in studies also focusing on Chinese youths.

Failure to accommodate trauma-related memories with existing self-capacities could disrupt emotional stability and induce tremendous distress, thus contributing to the development of posttraumatic stress symptoms (Briere, 1996). Nevertheless, the self-trauma model argues that these PTSD reactions are not merely symptoms of psychopathology but rather evolved mechanisms of repetitive activation and processing. In other words, intrusion could activate unresolved trauma memories in order to have them processed. As the activation and processing of trauma cues tends to produce psychological distress, if the distress accumulated to the extent that was beyond the victim's tolerance, he or she might display avoidance reactions to avoid or shut down further activation and processing for temporary protection of the self. However, once the distress was regulated to be tolerated, intrusion might again initiate the activation and processing of trauma. In such a circular manner, the intrusive and avoidance symptoms of PTSD alternate to repetitively activate and process suppressed trauma materials until completion. Given that the process of completion usually takes time, it is not surprising to find that 17%-20% of our adolescents still suffered probable PTSD even when their traumatic experiences occurred 3.63 to 4.35 years ago. These traumatized adolescents might have been processing their trauma-related memories via the aforementioned evolved defense mechanism.

Second, both our cross-sectional and longitudinal studies (i.e., Study 1, 2, and 3) confirmed significant associations between PTSD from past trauma and the positive and negative psychological outcomes (i.e., posttraumatic growth and psychiatric co-morbidity), although the directions of these relations seemed to be different between studies. Consistent with prior research regarding these three constructs, whilst PTSD from past trauma can be related to elevated psychiatric co-morbidity thus displaying a co-morbidity of these two disorders (Miller et al., 2004; Keane et al., 2007; Chung et al., 2017; Chung & Chen, 2017; Chen & Chung, 2016), the reverse could also happen under some circumstances (Creamer et al., 1992). With respect to posttraumatic growth, PTSD from past trauma was negatively associated with PTG in the cross-sectional study, but these two constructs were positively related in the subsequent longitudinal investigation. This inconsistency in the relationship between PTSD from past trauma and posttraumatic growth was also found in previous literature (Alisic et al., 2008; Barakat et al., 2006; Hafstad et al., 2010, 2011; Kilmer & Gil-Rivas, 2010; Kilmer et al., 2009; Laufer & Solomon, 2006; Laufer et al., 2009; Levine et al., 2008; Tian et al., 2016; Yu et al., 2010; Zhou et al., 2015; Du et al., 2018). Hence, the direct relationship between PTSD and PTG was somewhat unpredictable. As pointed out in Chapter 1, this might have some relation with the different levels of traumatic distress experienced by two different samples (Butler et al., 2005; Nelson, 2011; Tedeschi & Calhoun, 2004). Specifically, the distress in Study 2 might have been too overwhelming and beyond victims' tolerance, which undermined the emergence of PTG, whereas, the distress in Study 3 might have been at moderate levels which could facilitate the development of posttraumatic growth. In addition, although in Study 2 the direct relation between PTSD and PTG was negative, one must not only focus on this story. When we took account of trauma centrality and adaptive coping, these adolescents seemed to have certain resilient characteristics. Therefore, the directions of the associations between PTSD and psychological outcomes of psychiatric co-morbidity and growth could vary depending on the kind of psychological factors one is looking at.

Third, PTSD from past trauma robustly and positively predicted trauma centrality in both our retrospective and prospective studies. This is in line with the preceding literature (Ionio et al., 2018). As argued earlier, PTSD might have manifested itself via the symptoms of trauma centrality. Notwithstanding this, whether trauma centrality can mediate the impact of PTSD on psychological outcomes was unpredictable. Moreover, although coping (cognitive emotion regulation in this case) played some part in victims' fighting against trauma, it seemed to affect the development of posttraumatic growth only but not the development of psychiatric co-morbidity. Cognitive emotion regulation only mediated the effect of initial PTSD on subsequent PTG. As such, cognitive emotion regulation might have unique influences on the nurturance of posttraumatic growth. Together, these findings could suggest that trauma centrality and cognitive emotion regulation do not have generic mediational effects in the trauma research field. Rather, trauma centrality might be a psychological outcome itself and cognitive emotion regulation may only exert influences over specific psychological reactions.

Finally, our latent profile analysis explored how PTSD from past trauma could co-exist with cognitive emotion regulation and unresolved attachment to influence positive and negative psychological outcomes. Four latent profiles of adolescents were produced: the low trauma group, the adaptive coping group, the moderate trauma group, and the high trauma group. Aligned with the dose-response hypothesis (Dohrenwend & Dohrenwend, 1974; Henriksen et al., 2010; Johnson & Thompson, 2008), severely traumatized and highly unresolved youths (the high trauma group in this case) claimed the greatest severity of psychiatric co-morbid symptoms, whereas those moderately traumatized and moderately unresolved (the moderate trauma group in this case) reported moderate degrees of psychiatric co-morbidity, and those slightly traumatized and slightly unresolved (the low trauma group and adaptive coping group in this case) suffered the least. In terms of posttraumatic growth, adolescents in the high trauma group displayed the lowest levels while the adaptive coping group reported the highest. This corroborated the fundamental tenet of PTG (Tedeschi & Calhoun, 2004) and the protective role of adaptive CER on the development of posttraumatic growth (Garnefski et al., 2001; Garnefski et al., 2008).

Past traumatic experiences could affect victims' mental health and personal growth. This relationship between past trauma and psychological outcomes could be influenced by victims' coping and a combination of variables including attachment difficulties, but not necessarily by changes in self-concept. In other words, our past traumatic memories, past experiences with attachment figures, and what we do could affect psychological problems and growth. These past experiences are often out of victims' control, whereas coping tends to reflect conscious behaviors or activities and is usually within their control. Future studies could further examine the roles of losing control and having control on mental health outcomes in the aftermath of trauma. The impact of changes of oneself on psychological outcomes also needs more in-depth exploration, given its unpredictability on psychiatric co-morbidity and growth in the present thesis.

6.2 Implications

Our findings in the present thesis have significant clinical implications for posttraumatic adaptation and thriving among adolescents with a history of trauma exposure. Firstly, for mental health service centers, it would be favorable to screen for adolescents' PTSD symptoms, degree of trauma centrality, and adaptive and maladaptive coping. This information could promote tailored treatment for each individual. Secondly, by virtue of the significance of cognitive processing and emotion regulation in treating PTSD to facilitate posttraumatic growth, intervention programs targeting cognitive emotion regulation could be encouraged, especially aimed at strengthening patients' adaptive CER skills and decreasing the use of maladaptive ones. For policymakers and administrators, given the relatively high prevalence rates of trauma exposure and PTSD reactions among adolescents, it would be beneficial to promote psychoeducation at secondary schools on a regular basis. This psychoeducation would incorporate the aforesaid adaptive cognitive emotion regulation skills and could be carried out in various formats including lectures on posttraumatic growth, workshops on the concept of self, and emotion regulation training programs. They may provide opportunities for adolescents to process their trauma experiences, address issues associated with the dysfunctional aspect of the self, and learn or strengthen resilient skills of adaptive CER which enable adolescents to recover and thrive in the aftermath of trauma. Last but not least, when it comes to caregivers, guided by increasing evidence on the adverse effects of unresolved attachment on children's development and the benefits of secure attachment, parents should pay more attention to their parenting behaviors and the child's reactions, improve the quality of parent-child interactions, and provide a secure base from which the child could bravely explore the environment and develop a strong and healthy sense of self.

6.3   Future Research Directions

First, the present thesis consistently pointed to a positive association between PTSD from past trauma and trauma centrality, suggesting that trauma could challenge and alter victims' self-understanding,giving rise to a restructured traumatized self. This underscored the vulnerability of self-concept in the presence of trauma. However, trauma centrality was only one aspect of the traumatized self. Future studies may want to explore other aspects of the traumatized self such as the inert self, ego strength, and fragmented self proposed by the posttraumatic-self model (Wilson, 2006), which could extend our knowledge about the role of personal identity in adolescents' reactions to crises. Second, whilst trauma centrality was associated with psychiatric co-morbidity and posttraumatic growth in the first study, these relationships were not established in the second study of the present thesis. Such inconsistencies might be accounted for by differences in,for instance, demographic information, family background, and personality characteristics between the two cohorts of the first two studies. Accordingly, these factors might be taken into account in future research. Third, given that two types of cognitive emotion regulation skills failed to predict psychiatric co-morbidity in the present thesis,future researchers may want to take other kinds of coping into consideration, for instance, mindfulness, self-compassion, attentional control, and self-soothing, which might produce different results. Fourth, a randomized controlled trial of the aforementioned psychoeducation program could be carried out to look at the effect of these adaptive cognitive emotion regulation strategies in enhancing posttraumatic growth in the aftermath of trauma. Finally, given the important role attachment and cognitive-emotional coping played in adolescents' reactions to crises, it might be favorable to incorporate qualitative designs into future investigations so as to gain deeper insights into the psychological mechanisms under these two constructs.

6.4   Conclusions

The present thesis explored the influence of past trauma on positive and negative psychological outcomes and examined the roles of self-concept, coping, and attachment difficulties. Utilizing standardized measures and retrospective and prospective designs, the present thesis revealed findings that supported the self-trauma model and the models of PTG while extending these models with attachment theory. Following traumatic experiences, Chinese adolescents could suffer psychological distress on one hand and experience positive changes on the other. Trauma can also change adolescents' concept of self, but the impact of this traumatized self-structure on the aforesaid psychological outcomes cannot be predicted. Notwithstanding this, the coping of cognitive emotion regulation appeared to have unique effects on the development of positive changes but not on that of distress. Specifically, the adaptive pattern of thinking served as a protector, promoting the positive effect of trauma on growth, whereas the maladaptive one functioned like an inflictor impairing the nurturance of growth. In addition, attachment difficulties could co-exist with traumatic experiences and coping to influence the aforementioned positive and negative psychological reactions.

Bibliography

Abernathy, B. E. (2008). Who am I now? Helping trauma clients find meaning, wisdom, and a renewed sense of self. *Compelling counseling interventions: Celebrating VISTAS' fifth anniversary*, 199-208.

Aflakseir, A., & Manafi, F. (2018). Posttraumatic growth and its relationship with cognitive emotion regulation strategies in patients with multiple sclerosis in Shiraz, Iran. *Practice in Clinical Psychology*, 6(1), 57-62.

Afzali, M. H., Sunderland, M., Teesson, M., Carragher, N., Mills, K., Slade, T. (2017). A network approach to the co-morbidity between posttraumatic stress disorder and major depressive disorder: the role of overlapping symptoms. *Journal of Affective Disorders*, 208, 490-496.

Aguirre, M. (2008). *An examination of the role of meaning in posttraumatic growth following bereavement*. Doctoral dissertation, Auburn University.

Agustini, E. N., Asniar, I., & Matsuo, H. (2011). The prevalence of long-term post-traumatic stress symptoms among adolescents after the tsunami in Aceh. *Journal of Psychiatric and Mental Health Nursing*, 18(6), 543-549.

Ai, A. L., & Park, C. L. (2005). Possibilities of the positive following violence and trauma: Informing the coming decade of research. *Journal of Interpersonal Violence*, 20(2), 242-250.

Aldao A, Nolen-Hoeksema S, & Schweizer S. (2010). Emotion-regulation strategies across psychopathology: a meta-analytic review. *Clinical*

Psychology Review, 30(2), 217-37.

Aldwin, C. M., Levenson, M. R., & Spiro, A. (1994). Vulnerability and resilience to combat exposure: Can stress have lifelong effects? *Psychology and Aging*, 9(1), 34.

Algoe, S. B. (2005). *A relational account of gratitude: A positive emotion that strengthens interpersonal connections*. University of Virginia.

Alisic, E., van der Schoot, T. A. W., van Ginkel, J. R., Kleber, R. J. (2008). Looking beyond posttraumatic stress disorder in children: posttraumatic stress reactions, posttraumatic growth, and quality of life in a general population sample. *Journal of Clinical Psychiatry*, 69, 1455-1461.

American Psychiatric Association. (2013). *Diagnostic and Statistical Manual of Mental Disorders (DSM-5 ©)*. Arlington, US: American Psychiatric Publising.

Amone-P'Olak, K., Garnefski, N., & Kraaij, V. (2007). Adolescents caught between fires: Cognitive emotion regulation in response to war experiences in Northern Uganda. *Journal of adolescence*, 30(4), 655-669.

An, Y., Ding, X., & Fu, F. (2017). Personality and post-traumatic growth of adolescents 42 months after the Wenchuan earthquake: A mediated model. *Frontiers in Psychology*, 8, 2152.

An, Y., Huang, J., Chen, Y., & Deng, Z. (2019). Longitudinal cross-lagged relationships between posttraumatic stress disorder and depression in adolescents following the Yancheng tornado in China. *Psychological trauma: theory, research, practice and policy*, 11(7), 760-766.

An, Y., Yuan, G., Zhang, N., Xu, W., Liu, Z., & Zhou, F. (2018). Longitudinal cross-lagged relationships between mindfulness, posttraumatic stress symptoms, and posttraumatic growth in adolescents following the Yancheng tornado in China. *Psychiatry*

Research, 266, 334-340.

Ang, R. P., & Huan, V. S. (2006). Relationship between academic stress and suicidal ideation: testing for depression as a mediator using multiple regression. *Child Psychiatry and Human Development*, 37 (2), 133-143.

Arata, C. M., Langhinrichsen-Rohling, J., Bowers, D., & O'Farrill-Swails, L. (2005). Single versus multi-type maltreatment: an examination of the long-term effects of child abuse. *Journal of Aggression Maltreatment & Trauma*, 11, 29-52.

Armour, C., Fried, E. I., Deserno, M. K., Tsai, J., Pietrzak, R. H. (2017). A network analysis of DSM-5 posttraumatic stress disorder symptoms and correlates in U. S. military veterans. *Journal of Anxiety Disorders*, 45, 49-59.

Asarnow, J., Glynn, S., Pynoos, R. S., Nahum, J., Guthrie, D., Cantwell, D. P., Franklin, B. (1999). When the earth stops shaking: Earthquake sequelae among children diagnosed for pre-earthquake psychopathology. *Journal of the American Academy of Child and Adolescent Psychiatry*, 38, 1016-1023.

Au, T. A., Dickstein, B. D., Comera, J. S., Salters-Pedneault, K., & Litz, B. T. (2013). Co-occurring posttraumatic stress and depression symptoms after sexual assault: A latent profile analysis. *Journal of Affective Disorders*, 49, 209-216.

Auerbach, R. P., Claro, A., Abela, J. R., Zhu, X., & Yao, S. (2010). Understanding risky behavior engagement amongst Chinese adolescents. *Cognitive Therapy and Research*, 34(2), 159-167.

Barakat, L. P., Alderfer, M. A., & Kazak, A. E. (2006). Posttraumatic growth in adolescent survivors of cancer and their mothers and fathers. *Journal of Pediatric Psychology*, 31, 413-419.

Baron, P. (1986). Egocentrism and depressive symptomatology in adolescents. *Journal of Adolescent Research*, 1(4), 431-437.

Bartels, L., Berliner, L., Holt, T., Jensen, T., Jungbluth, N., Plener, P., ... Sachser, C. (2019). The importance of the DSM-5 PTSD symptoms of cognitions and mood in traumatized children and adolescents: Two network approaches. *Journal of Child Psychology and Psychiatry*, 60, 545-554.

Barton, S., Boals, A., & Knowles, L. (2013). Thinking about trauma: the unique contributions of event centrality and posttraumatic cognitions in predicting PTSD and posttraumatic growth. *Journal of Traumatic Stress*, 26, 718-726.

Barry, C. T., Reiter, S. R., Anderson, A. C., Schoessler, M. L., & Sidoti, C. L. (2019). "Let me take another selfie": Further examination of the relation between narcissism, self-perception, and Instagram posts. *Psychology of Popular Media Culture*, 8(1), 22.

Beck, A. T., Brown, G., Steer, R. A., Eidelson, J. I., Riskind, J. H. (1987). Differentiating anxiety and depression: a test of the cognitive content-specificity hypothesis. *Journal of Abnormal Psychology*, 96(3), 179.

Beck, R., & Perkins, T. S. (2001). Cognitive content-specificity for anxiety and depression: A meta-analysis. *Cognitive Therapy and Research*, 25(6), 651-663.

Beck, A. T., Steer, R. A., & Brown, G. K. (1996). *Beck depression inventory-II (BDI-II)* (Vol. 10, p. s15327752jpa6703_13). Pearson.

Belle, D. (1991). Gender differences in the social moderators of stress. In A. Monat & R. S. Lazarus (Eds.), *Stress and coping: Ananthology* (pp. 258-274). New York: Columbia University Press.

Bellet, B. W., Jones, P. J., Neimeyer, R. A., Mcnally, R. J. (2018). Bereavement outcomes as causal systems: a network analysis of the co-occurrence of complicated grief and posttraumatic growth. *Clinical Psychological Science*, 6(6), 797-809.

Bellizzi, K. M. , & Blank, T. O. (2006). Predicting posttraumatic growth in breast cancer survivors. *Health Psychology*, 25(1), 47-56.

Benight, C. C. , Shoji, K. , & Delahanty, D. L. (2017). Self-regulation shift theory: a dynamic systems approach to traumatic stress. *Journal of Traumatic Stress*, 30(4), 333-342.

Benzein, E. G. , & Berg, A. C. (2005). The level of and relation between hope, hopelessness and fatigue in patients and family members in palliative care. *Palliative Medicine*, 19(3), 234-240.

Berntsen, D. , & Rubin, D. C. (2006). The centrality of event scale: a measure of integrating a trauma into one's identity and its relation to post-traumatic stress disorder symptoms. *Behaviour Research and Therapy*, 44, 219-231.

Blix, I. , Birkeland, M. S. , Hansen, M. B. , & Heir, T. (2015). Posttraumatic growth and centrality of event: A longitudinal study in the aftermath of the 2011 Oslo bombing. *Psychological Trauma : Theory, Research, Practice, and Policy*, 7(1), 18.

Boals, A. , & Schuettler, D. (2011). A double-edged sword: event centrality, PTSD and posttraumatic growth. *Applied Cognitive Psychology*, 25, 817-822.

Boals, A. , & Schuler, K. L. (2018). Reducing reports of illusory posttraumatic growth: A revised version of the Stress-Related Growth Scale (SRGS-R). *Psychological Trauma : Theory, Research, Practice, and Policy*, 10(2), 190.

Boisseau, C. L. , Thompson-Brenner, H. , Eddy, K. T. , & Satir, D. A. (2009). Impulsivity and personality variables in adolescents with eating disorders. *The Journal of Nervous and Mental Disease*, 197, 4.

Bokszczanin, A. (2007). PTSD symptoms in children and adolescents 28 months after a flood: Age and gender differences. *Journal of Traumatic Stress*, 20(3), 347-351.

Bower, J. E., Kemeny, M. E., Taylor, S. E., & Fahey, J. L. (1998). Cognitive processing, discovery of meaning, CD4 decline, and AIDS-related mortality among bereaved HIV-seropositive men. *Journal of Consulting and Clinical Psychology*, 66, 979-986.

Bowlby, J. (1973). *Attachment and Loss, Vol. 2: Separation-anxiety and anger.* New York: Basic Books.

Bowlby, J. (1980). *Attachment and loss: vol. 3. Loss: sadness and depression.* New York: Basic Books.

Bowlby, J. (1982). Attachment and loss: retrospect and prospect. *American Journal of Orthopsychiatry*, 52(4), 664.

Brady, K. T., Killeen, T. K., Brewerton, T., & Lucerini, S. (2000). Co-morbidity of psychiatric disorders and posttraumatic stress disorder. *The Journal of Clinical Psychiatry*, 61(Suppl 7), 22-32.

Brancu, M., Mann-Wrobel, M., Beckham, J. C., Wagner, H. R., Elliott, A., Robbins, A. T., ... & Runnals, J. J. (2016). Subthreshold posttraumatic stress disorder: A meta-analytic review of DSM-IV prevalence and a proposed DSM-5 approach to measurement. *Psychological trauma: theory, research, practice, and policy*, 8(2), 222-232.

Breslau, N., Chilcoat, H. D., Kessler, R. C., & Davis, G. C. (1999). Previous exposure to trauma and PTSD effects of subsequent trauma: Results from the Detroit Area Survey of Trauma. *American Journal of Psychiatry*, 156, 902-907.

Breslau, N., Lucia, V. C., & Davis, G. C. (2004). Partial PTSD versus full PTSD: an empirical examination of associated impairment.

Psychological medicine, 34(7), 1205-1214.

Breslau, N. , Wilcox, H. C. , Storr, C. L. , Lucia, V. C. , & Anthony, J. C. (2004). Trauma exposure and posttraumatic stress disorder: a study of youths in urban America. *Journal of Urban Health : Bulletin of the New York Academy of Medicine*, 81(4): 530-544.

Brewin, C. R. , Dalgleish, T. , & Joseph, S. (1996). A dual representation theory of posttraumatic stress disorder. *Psychological review*, 103 (4), 670.

Briere, J. (1992). *Child Abuse Trauma : Theory and Treatment of the Lasting Effects*. Newbury Park, CA: Sage.

Briere, J. (1996). *Therapy for Adults Molested as Children*, Second Edition, Expanded and Revised. New York: Springer Publishing Co.

Briere, J. (2002). Treating adult survivors of severe childhood abuse and neglect: further development of an integrative model. In J. E. B. Myers, L. Berliner, J. Briere, C. T. Hendrix, C. Jenny, & T. A. Reid (Eds.), *The APSAC handbook on child maltreatment* (2nd ed. , pp. 175-203). Sage Publications, Inc.

Briere, J. , & Elliott, D. (1994). Immediate and long-term impacts of child sexual abuse. *The Future of Children*, 4(2), 54-69.

Bringmann, L. F. , Lemmens, L. H. J. M. , Huibers, M. J. H. , Borsboom, D. , & Tuerlinckx, F. (2015). Revealing the dynamic network structure of the Beck Depression Inventory-Ⅱ. *Psychological Medicine*, 45, 747-757.

Brooks, M. , Graham-Kevan, N. , Lowe, M. , & Robinson, S. (2017). Rumination, event centrality, and perceived control as predictors of post-traumatic growth and distress: the cognitive growth and stress model. *British Journal of Clinical Psychology*, 56, 286-302.

Browne, A. , & Finkelhor, D. (1986). Impact of child sexual abuse: A review of the research. *Psychological Bulletin*, 99(1), 66-77.

Butler, L. D. , Blasey, C. M. , Garlan, R. W. , McCaslin, S. E. , Azarow, J. , Chen, X. H. ,... & Kraemer, H. C. (2005). Posttraumatic growth following the terrorist attacks of September 11, 2001: Cognitive, coping, and trauma symptom predictors in an internet convenience sample. *Traumatology*, 11(4), 247-267.

Calhoun, L. G. , & Tedeschi, R. G. (1991). Perceiving benefits in traumatic events: Some issues for practicing psychologists. *Journal of Training & Practice in Professional Psychology*, 5(1), 45-52.

Calhoun, L. G. , & Tedeschi, R. G. (2006). The foundations of posttraumatic growth: An expanded framework. *Handbook of posttraumatic growth: Research and practice* (pp. 3-23). Lawrence Erlbaum Associates Publishers.

Cann, A. , Calhoun, L. G. , Tedeschi, R. G. , & Solomon, D. T. (2010). Posttraumatic growth and depreciation as independent experiences and predictors of well-being. *Journal of Loss and Trauma*, 15, 151-166.

Cao, X. , Wang, L. , Cao, C. , Fang, R. , Chen, C. , Hall, B. J. , & Elhai, J. D. (2019). Sex differences in global and local connectivity of adolescent posttraumatic stress disorder symptoms. *Journal of child psychology and psychiatry, and allied disciplines*, 60(2), 216-224.

Cao, X. , Wang, L. , Cao, C. , & Zhang, J. (2015). The phenotypic model of posttraumatic stress disorder symptom dimensionality [Chinese]. *Journal of Beijing Normal University (Social Sciences)*, 6, 87-99.

Carliner, H. , Keyes, K. M. , McLaughlin, K. A. , Meyers, J. L. , Dunn, E. C. , & Martins, S. S. (2016). Childhood trauma and illicit drug use in adolescence: A population-based national comorbidity survey replication-adolescent supplement study. *Journal of The American Academy of Child & Adolescent Psychiatry*, 55(8), 791-708.

Carmassi, C. , Akiskal, H. S. , Yong, S. S. , Stratta, P. , Calderani, E. ,

Massimetti, E. ,... & Dell'Osso, L. (2013). Post-traumatic stress disorder in DSM-5: estimates of prevalence and criteria comparison versus DSM-Ⅳ-TR in a non-clinical sample of earthquake survivors. *Journal of Affective Disorders*,151(3),843-848.

Carver,C. S. ,& Scheier,M. F. (1998). *On the self-regulation of behavior*. New York: Cambridge University Press.

Casey,B. J. (2015). Beyond simple models of self-control to circuit-based accounts of adolescent behavior. *Annual Review of Psychology*, 66, 295-319.

Cervantes, R. C. , Cardoso, J. B. , Goldbach J. T. (2015). Examining differences in culturally based stress among clinical and nonclinical Hispanic adolescents. *Cultural diversity & ethnic minority psychology*,21(3),458-467.

Chan,K. L. (2013). Victimization and poly-victimization among school-aged Chinese adolescents: Prevalence and associations with health. *Preventive medicine*,56(3-4),207-210.

Charles, N. E. , Reiter, S. R. , & Barry, C. T. (2019). The extent and correlates of stressors experienced by at-risk youths in a military-style residential program. *Journal of Child and Family Studies*, 28, 1313-1325.

Chen,Z. S. , & Chung, M. C. (2016). The relationship between gender, posttraumatic stress disorder from past trauma, alexithymia and psychiatric co-morbidity in Chinese adolescents: a moderated mediational analysis. *Psychiatric Quarterly*,87(4),689-701.

Chen,T. Y. ,Chou,Y. C. ,Tzeng,N. S. ,Chang,H. A. ,Kuo,S. C. ,Pan,P. Y. , Yeh, Y. W. , Yeh,C. B. , & Mao,W. C. (2015a). Effects of a selective educational system on fatigue, sleep problems, daytime sleepiness, and depression among senior high school adolescents in

Taiwan. *Neuropsychiatric disease and treatment*, 11, 741-750.

Chen, S. H., Lin, Y. H., Tseng, H. M., & Wu, Y. C. (2002). Posttraumatic stress reactions in children and adolescents one year after the 1999 Taiwan Chi-Chi earthquake. *Journal of the Chinese Institute of Engineers*, 25, 597-608.

Chen, J., Zhou, X., Zeng, M., & Wu, X. (2015b). Post-traumatic stress symptoms and posttraumatic growth: evidence from a longitudinal study following an earthquake disaster. *PLoS One* 10 (6), e0127241.

Choi, K. W., Batchelder, A. W., Ehlinger, P. P., Safren, S. A., & O'Cleirigh, C. (2017). Applying network analysis to psychological co-morbidity and health behavior: Depression, PTSD, and sexual risk in sexual minority men with trauma histories. *Journal of consulting and clinical psychology*, 85(12), 1158-1170.

Chung, M. C., AlQarni, N., Muhairi, S. A., & Mitchell, B. (2017). The relationship between trauma centrality, self-efficacy, posttraumatic stress and psychiatric co-morbidity among Syrian refugees: Is gender a moderator? *Journal of psychiatric research*, 94, 107-115.

Chung, M. C., & Chen, Z. S. (2017). Child abuse and psychiatric co-morbidity among Chinese adolescents: Emotional processing as mediator and PTSD from past trauma as moderator. *Child Psychiatry & Human Development*, 48(4), 610-618.

Chung, M. C., & Chen, Z. S. (2020). Gender differences in child abuse, emotional processing difficulties, alexithymia, psychological symptoms and behavioral problems among Chinese adolescents. *Psychiatric quarterly*, 91(2), 321-332.

Chung, M. C., Dennis, I., Easthope, Y., Werrett, J., & Farmer, S. (2005). A multiple-indicator multiple-cause model for posttraumatic stress reactions: personality, coping, and maladjustment. *Psychosomatic*

Medicine, 67(2), 251-259.

Chung, M. C. , Shakra, M. , AlQarni, N. , AlMazrouei, M. , Mazrouei, S. A. , & Hashimi, S. A. (2018). Posttraumatic stress among Syrian refugees: trauma exposure characteristics, trauma centrality, and emotional suppression. *Psychiatry*, 81(1), 54-70.

Ciesla, J. A. , & Roberts, J. E. (2007). Rumination, negative cognition, and their interactive effects on depressed mood. *Emotion*, 7(3), 555-565.

Clark, D. B. , Lesnick, L. , & Hegedus, A. M. (1997). Traumas and other adverse life events in adolescents with alcohol abuse and dependence. *Journal of the American Academy of Child and Adolescent Psychiatry*, 36(12), 1744-1751.

Clay, R. , Knibbs, J. , & Joseph, S. (2009). Measurement of posttraumatic growth in young people: A review. *Clinical Child Psychology and Psychiatry*, 14(3), 411-422.

Cohen, J. A. (1998). Practice parameters for the assessment and treatment of children and adolescents with posttraumatic stress disorder. *Journal of the American Academy of Child and Adolescent Psychiatry*, 37 (10 Suppl), 4s-26s.

Cohen, J. R. , Hankin, B. L. , Gibb, B. E. , Hammen, C. , Hazel, N. A. , Ma, D. ,... & Abela, J. R. (2013). Negative attachment cognitions and emotional distress in mainland Chinese adolescents: A prospective multiwave test of vulnerability-stress and stress generation models. *Journal of Clinical Child & Adolescent Psychology*, 42(4), 531-544.

Cole, D. A. , & Maxwell, S. E. (2003). Testing mediational models with longitudinal data: questions and tips in the use of structural equation modeling. *Journal of abnormal psychology*, 112 (4), 558-577.

Conway, M. A. , & Pleydell-Pearce, C. W. (2000). The construction of autobiographical memories in the self-memory system. *Psychological review*,107(2),261-288.

Copeland, W. E. , Keeler, G. , Angold, A. , & Costello, E. J. (2007). Traumatic events and posttraumatic stress in childhood. *Archives of general psychiatry*,64(5),577-584

Costa Jr,P. T. , & McCrae,R. R. (1992). Four ways five factors are basic. *Personality and Individual Differences*,13(6),653-665.

Creamer,M. , Burgess, P. P. , & McFarlane, A. C. (2001). Post-traumatic stress disorder:Findings from the Australian National Survey of Mental Health and Well-Being. *Psychological Medicine: A Journal of Research in Psychiatry and the Allied Sciences*,31(7),1237-1247.

Creamer,M. , Burgess, P. , & Pattison, P. (1992). Reaction to trauma: A cognitive processing model. *Journal of abnormal psychology*,101(3), 452-459.

Cramer, A. O. , Waldorp, L. J. , van der Maas, H. L. , & Borsboom, D. (2010). Co-morbidity: A network perspective. *Behavioral and Brain Sciences*,33(2-3),137-193.

Creighton, S. J. (2004). *Prevalence and incidence of child abuse: International comparisons*. NSPCC Information Briefings.

Cryder,C. H. ,Kilmer,R. P. ,Tedeschi,R. G. , & Calhoun,L. G. (2006). An exploratory study of posttraumatic growth in children following a natural disaster. *American Journal of Orthopsychiatry*,76(1),65-69.

Csardi,G. , & Nepusz,T. (2006). The igraph software package for complex network research. *InterJournal*,*Complex Systems*,1695.

Cunha,M. , Xavier, A. , Matos, M. , & Faria, D. (2015). O impacto das memórias de vergonha na adolescência: A Escala da Centralidade do Acontecimento (CES) [The impact of shame memories in adolescence: the Centrality of Event Scale (CES)]. *Análise Psicológica*,3,1-14.

d'Acremont,M. , & Van der Linden,M. (2007). How is impulsivity related to depression in adolescence? Evidence from a French validation of the cognitive emotion regulation questionnaire. *Journal of adolescence*, 30 (2), 271-282.

Darnell, D., Flaster, A., Hendricks, K., Kerbrat, A., & Comtois, K. A. (2019). Adolescent clinical populations and associations between trauma and behavioral and emotional problems. *Psychological Trauma: Theory, Research, Practice, and Policy*, 11(3), 266-273.

Davis, L., & Siegel, L. J. (2000). Posttraumatic stress disorder in children and adolescents: A review and analysis. *Clinical child and family psychology review*, 3(3), 135-154.

De Haan, A., Landolt, M. A., Fried, E. I., Kleinke, K., Alisic, E., Bryant, R.,... & Meiser-Stedman, R. (2020). Dysfunctional posttraumatic cognitions, posttraumatic stress and depression in children and adolescents exposed to trauma: a network analysis. *Journal of Child Psychology and Psychiatry*, 61(1), 77-87.

Dekel, S., Ein-Dor, T., & Solomon, Z. (2012). Posttraumatic growth and posttraumatic distress: a longitudinal study. *Psychological Trauma Theory Research Practice and Policy*, 4(1), 94-101.

Deykin, E. Y., & Buka, S. L. (1997). Prevalence and risk factors for posttraumatic stress disorder among chemically dependent adolescents. *The American Journal of Psychiatry*, 154(6), 752-757.

Djelantik, A. A. A. M. J., Robinaugh, D. J., Kleber, R. J., Smid, G. E., & Boelen, P. A. (2019). Symptomatology following loss and trauma: latent class and network analyses of prolonged grief disorder, posttraumatic stress disorder, and depression in a treatment-seeking trauma-exposed sample. *Depression & Anxiety*, 37(1), 26-34.

Dohrenwend, B. S., & Dohrenwend, B. P. (1974). *Stressful life events: Their nature and effects*. Oxford: John Wiley & Sons.

Doorley,J. , Williams,C. , Mallard, T. , Esposito-Smythers,C. & McGeary, John. (2017). Sexual trauma, the dopamine D4 receptor, and suicidal ideation among hospitalized adolescents: A preliminary investigation. *Archives of Suicide Research*,21(2),279-292.

Du,B. L. ,Ma,X. Z. ,Ou,X. C. ,Jin,Y. ,Ren,P. W. , & Li,J. (2018). The prevalence of posttraumatic stress in adolescents eight years after the Wenchuan earthquake. *Psychiatry research*,262,262-269.

Elkind,D. (1967). Egocentrism in adolescence. *Child development*,38(4), 1025-1034.

Elkind, D. (1985). Cognitive development and adolescent disabilities. *Journal of Adolescent Health Care*,6(2),84-89.

Elklit, A. (2002). Victimization and PTSD in a Danish national youth probability sample. *Journal of the American Academy of Child and Adolescent Psychiatry*,41(2),174-181.

Elklit, A. , & Petersen, T. (2008). Exposure to traumatic events among adolescents in four nations. *Torture*,18 (1),2-11.

Engel, C. C. (2004). Somatization and multiple idiopathic physical symptoms: Relationship to traumatic events and posttraumatic stress disorder. In P. P. Schnurr & B. L. Green (Eds.), *Trauma and health, physical health consequences of exposure to extreme stress* (pp. 191-215). Washington,D. C. : American Psychological Association.

Enright,R. , Lapsley,D. , and Shukla,D. (1979). Adolescent egocentrism in early and late adolescence. *Adolescence*,14,687-695.

Enright, R. D. , Shukla, D. G. , & Lapsley, D. K. (1980). Adolescent egocentrism-sociocentrism and self-consciousness. *Journal of youth and adolescence*,9(2),101-116.

Epskamp, S. , Borsboom, D. , Fried, E. I. , 2018. Estimating psychological networks and their accuracy: a tutorial paper. *Behavior research methods*,50(1),195-212.

Epskamp, S. , Cramer, A. O. , Waldorp, L. J. , Schmittmann, V. D. , & Borsboom,D. (2012). qgraph: Network visualizations of relationships in psychometric data. *Journal of Statistical Software*,48 (4),1-18.

Epskamp, S. , & Fried, E. I. (2018). A tutorial on regularized partial correlation networks. *Psychological Methods*,23 (4),617-634.

Epskamp,S. ,Rhemtulla,M. ,& Borsboom,D. (2017). Generalized network psychometrics: Combining network and latent variable models. *Psychometrika*,82(4),904-927.

Erikson,E. H. (1968). *Identity:Youth and crisis*. New York:Norton.

Fan,C. ,Chu,X. ,Wang,M. ,& Zhou,Z. (2016). Interpersonal stressors in the schoolyard and depressive symptoms among Chinese adolescents: The mediating roles of rumination and co-rumination. *School Psychology International*,37(6),664-679.

Fang,X. ,Fry,D. A. ,Ji,K. ,Finkelhor,D. ,Chen,J. ,Lannen,P. ,et al. (2015). The burden of child maltreatment in China: A systematic review. *Bulletin of the World Health Organization*,93(3),176-185.

Farina,A. S. ,Holzer,K. J. ,DeLisi,M. ,& Vaughn,M. G. (2018). Childhood trauma and psychopathic features among juvenile offenders. *International journal of offender therapy and comparative criminology*,62(14),4359-4380.

Finney,S. J. ,& DiStefano,C. (2006). Nonnormal and categorical data in structural equation modeling. In: Hancock, G. R. , Mueller, R. O. (Eds.), *Structural Equation Modeling : A Second Course*. Greenwich, CT:IAP.

Fitzgerald,J. M. (1988). Vivid memories and the reminiscence phenomenon: the role of a self-narrative. *Human Development*,31(5),261-273.

Fitzgerald,J. M. ,Berntsen,D. ,& Broadbridge,C. L. (2016). The influences of event centrality in memory models of PTSD. *Applied Cognitive Psychology*, 30, 10-21.

Frankenberger, K. D. (2004). Adolescent egocentrism, risk perceptions, and sensation seeking among smoking and nonsmoking youth. *Journal of Adolescent Research*, 19(5), 576-590.

Fried, E. I. (2015). Problematic assumptions have slowed down depression research: Why symptoms, not syndromes are the way forward. *Frontiers of Psychology*, 6, 1-11.

Friedman, J., Hastie, T., & Tibshirani, R. (2008). Sparse inverse covariance estimation with the graphical lasso. *Biostatistics*, 9(3), 432-441.

Friedman, M. J., Resick, P. A., Bryant, R. A., & Brewin, C. R. (2011). Considering PTSD for DSM-5. *Depression and anxiety*, 28 (9), 750-769.

Fredrickson, B. L. (2001). The role of positive emotions in positive psychology: The broaden-and-build theory of positive emotions. *The American psychologist*, 56(3), 218-226.

Fredrickson, B. L., & Branigan, C. (2005). Positive emotions broaden the scope of attention and thought-action repertoires. *Cognition & Emotion*, 19(3), 313-332.

Fredrickson, B. L., & Cohn, M. A. (2008). Positive emotions. In Lewis, M., Haviland-Jones, J. M., & Barrett, L. F. (Eds.). (2010). *Handbook of emotions (Third ed.)*. New York: the Guilford Press.

Freyd, J. (1994). Betrayal trauma: Traumatic amnesia as an adaptive response to childhood abuse. *Ethics & Behavior*, 4, 307-329.

Friedman, M., Keane, T., & Resick, P. (2007). *Handbook of PTSD: Science and Practice*. New York: the Guilford Press.

Fruchterman, T. M., & Reingold, E. M. (1991). Graph drawing by force-directed placement. *Software: Practice and Experience*, 21 (11),

1129-1164.

Frueh, B. C. , Elhai, J. D. , & Acierno, R. (2010). The future of posttraumatic stress disorder in the DSM. *Psychological Injury and Law* , 3, 260-270.

Fuligni, A. J. , Telzer, E. H. , Bower, J. , Cole, S. W. , Kiang, L. , & Irwin, M. R. (2009). A preliminary study of daily interpersonal stress and C-reactive protein levels among adolescents from Latin American and European backgrounds. *Psychosomatic medicine* , 71(3), 329.

Gaines Jr. , S. O. , Marelich, W. D. , Bledsoe, K. L. , Steers, W. N. , Henderson, M. C. , Granrose, C. S. , et al. (1997). Links between race/ethnicity and cultural values as mediated by racial/ethnic identity and moderated by gender. *Journal of personality and social psychology* , 72 (6), 1460-1476.

Galea, S. , Nandi, A. , & Vlahov, D. (2005). The epidemiology of post-traumatic stress disorder after disasters. *Epidemiologic reviews* , 27(1), 78-91.

Garber, J. , Weiss, B. , & Shanley, N. (1993). Cognitions, depressive symptoms, and development in adolescents. *Journal of abnormal psychology* , 102(1), 47-57.

Garland, E. L. , Carter, K. , & Howard, M. O. (2011). Prevalence, correlates, and characteristics of gasoline inhalation among high-risk youth: Associations with suicidal ideation, self-medication, and antisociality. *Klinik Psikofarmakoloji Bülteni-Bulletin of Clinical Psychopharmacology* , 21(2), 105-113.

Garland, E. L. , Farb, N. A. , R. Goldin, P. , & Fredrickson, B. L. (2015). Mindfulness broadens awareness and builds eudaimonic meaning: A process model of mindful positive emotion regulation. *Psychological Inquiry* , 26(4), 293-314.

Garland, E. L. , Pettus-Davis, C. , & Howard, M. O. (2013). Self-medication among traumatized youth: structural equation modeling of pathways between trauma history, substance misuse, and psychological distress. *Journal of behavioral medicine*, 36(2), 175-185.

Garnefski, N. , Kraaij, V. , & Spinhoven, P. (2001). Negative life events, cognitive emotion regulation and depression. *Personality and Individual Differences*, 30(8), 1311-1327.

Garnefski, N. , & Kraaij, V. (2006). Cognitive emotion regulation questionnaire—development of a short 18-item version (CERQ-short). *Personality and Individual Differences*, 41(6), 1045-1053.

Garnefski, N. , Kraaij, V. , Schroevers, M. J. , & Somsen, G. A. (2008). Post-traumatic growth after a myocardial infarction: a matter of personality, psychological health, or cognitive coping? *Journal of Clinical Psychology in Medical Settings*, 15(4), 270-277.

Ge, Fenfen, Yuan, Minlan, Li, Y. , Zhang, J. , & Zhang, W. (2019). Changes in the network structure of posttraumatic stress disorder symptoms at different time points among youth survivors: A network analysis. *Journal of Affective Disorders*, 259, 288-295.

Ghazali, S. R. , & Chen, Y. Y. (2018). Reliability, concurrent validity, and cutoff score of PTSD Checklist (PCL-5) for the Diagnostic and Statistical Manual of Mental Disorders, among Malaysian adolescents. *Traumatology*, 24(4), 280-287.

Ghazali, S. R. , Elklit, A. , Balang, R. V. , Sultan, M. A. , & Kana, K. (2014). Preliminary findings on lifetime trauma prevalence and PTSD symptoms among adolescents in Sarawak Malaysia. *Asian journal of psychiatry*, 11, 45-49.

Goldberg, D. , & Bridges, K. W. (1987). Screening for psychiatric illness in general practice: the general practitioner versus the screening questionnaire. *The Journal of the Royal College of General*

Practitioners, 37, 15-18.

Goldberg, D., & Hillier, V. (1979). A scaled version of the general health questionnaire. *Psychological medicine*, 9(1), 139-145.

Golino, H. F. (2016). *EGA package*. Github.com. http://github.com/hfgolino/EGA

Golino, H. F., & Demetriou, A. (2017). Estimating the dimensionality of intelligence like data using Exploratory Graph Analysis. *Intelligence*, 62, 54-70.

Golino, H. F., & Epskamp, S. (2017). Exploratory graph analysis: a new approach for estimating the number of dimensions in psychological research. *PLOS One* 12(6), e0174035.

Gooding, II. C., Millirenc, C., Austin, S. B., Sheridan, M. A., & McLaughlin, K. A. (2015). Exposure to violence in childhood is associated with higher body mass index in adolescence. *Child Abuse & Neglect*, 50, 151-158.

Gootzeit, J., & Markon, K. (2011). Factors of PTSD: differential specificity and external correlates. *Clinical psychology review*, 31(6), 993-1003.

Greenberg, M. A. (1995). Cognitive Processing of Traumas: the role of intrusive thoughts and reappraisals. *Journal of Applied Social Psychology*, 25(14), 1262-1296.

Greenwald, R. (2002). The role of trauma in conduct disorder. *Journal of Aggression, Maltreatment, & Trauma*, 6, 5-23.

Groleau, J. M., Calhoun, L. G., Cann, A., & Tedeschi, R. G. (2013). The role of centrality of events in posttraumatic distress and posttraumatic growth. *Psychological Trauma Theory Research Practice and Policy*, 5, 477-483.

Gross, J. J. (1998). Antecedent- and response-focused emotion regulation: divergent consequences for experience, expression, and physiology.

Journal of Personality and Social Psychology, 74(1), 224-237.

Gross, J. J., & Muñoz, R. F. (1995). Emotion regulation and mental health. *Clinical psychology: Science and practice*, 2(2), 151-164.

Gunn, H. E., Troxel, W. M., Hall, M. H., & Buysse, D. J. (2014). Interpersonal distress is associated with sleep and arousal in insomnia and good sleepers. *Journal of psychosomatic research*, 76(3), 242-248.

Gupta, M. A. (2006). Somatization disorders in dermatology. *International Review of Psychiatry*, 18(1), 41-47.

Gupta, M. A., Lanius, R. A., & van der Kolk, B. A. (2005). Psychologic trauma, posttraumatic stress disorder, and dermatology. *Dermatologic Clinics*, 23(4), 649-656.

Gustafsson, H., Doyle, C., Gilchrist, M., Werner, E., & Monk, C. (2017). Maternal abuse history and reduced fetal heart rate variability: Abuse-related sleep disturbance is a mediator. *Development and Psychopathology*, 29(3), 1023-1034.

Gyurak, A., Gross, J. J., & Etkin, A. (2011). Explicit and implicit emotion regulation: A dual-process framework. *Cognition and emotion*, 25(3), 400-412.

Hafstad, G. S., Gil-Rivas, V., Kilmer, R. P., & Raeder, S. (2010). Parental adjustment, family functioning, and posttraumatic growth among Norwegian children and adolescents following a natural disaster. *The American journal of orthopsychiatry*, 80(2), 248-257.

Hafstad, G. S., Kilmer, R. P., & Gil-Rivas, V. (2011). Posttraumatic adjustment and posttraumatic growth among Norwegian children and adolescents to the 2004 Tsunami. *Psychological Trauma: Theory, Research, Practice, and Policy*, 3, 130-138.

Hagenaars, M. A., & van Minnen, A. (2010). Posttraumatic growth in exposure therapy for PTSD. *Journal of Trauma and Stress*, 23(4),

504-508.

Hankin, B. L. , & Abramson, L. Y. (2001). Development of gender differences in depression: An elaborated cognitive vulnerability-transactional stress theory. *Psychological Bulletin*, 127(6), 773-796.

Hanley, A. W. , Garland, E. L. , & Tedeschi, R. G. (2017). Relating dispositional mindfulness, contemplative practice, and positive reappraisal with posttraumatic cognitive coping, stress, and growth. *Psychological Trauma: Theory, Research, Practice, and Policy*, 9(5), 526-536.

Hanley, A. W. , Peterson, G. W. , Canto, A. I. , & Garland, E. L. (2015). The relationship between mindfulness and posttraumatic growth with respect to contemplative practice engagement. *Mindfulness*, 6(3), 654-662.

Harari, D. , Bakermans-Kranenburg, M. J. , De Kloet, C. S. , Geuze, E. , Vermetten, E. , Westenberg, H. G. M. , & Van IJzendoorn, M. H. (2009). Attachment representations in Dutch veterans with and without deployment-related PTSD. *Attachment & Human Development*, 11(6), 515-536.

Hau, K. T. , & Marsh, H. W. (2004). The use of item parcels in structural equation modeling: nonnormal data and small sample sizes. *The British journal of mathematical and statistical psychology*, 57(Pt 2), 327-351.

Heckhausen, J. , Wrosch, C. , & Schulz, R. (2010). A motivational theory of life-span development. *Psychological Review*, 117(1), 32-60.

Helgeson, V. S. , Reynolds, K. A. , & Tomich, P. L. (2006). A meta-analytic review of benefit finding and growth. *Journal of consulting and clinical psychology*, 74(5), 797-816.

Henriksen, C. A. , Bolton, J. M. , & Sareen, J. (2010). The psychological impact of terrorist attacks: Examining dose-response relationship between exposure to 9/11 and Axis I mental disorders. *Depression and Anxiety*, 27(11), 993-1000.

Hirooka, K., Fukahori, H., Ozawa, M., & Akita, Y. (2017). Differences in posttraumatic growth and grief reactions among adolescents by relationship with the deceased. *Journal of Advanced Nursing*, 73(4), 955-965.

Hobfoll, S. E. (1989). Conservation of resources: A new attempt at conceptualizing stress. *American Psychologist*, 44(3), 513-524.

Hobfoll, S. E., Hall, B. J., Canetti-Nisim, D., Galea, S., Johnson, R. J., & Palmieri, P. A. (2007). Refining our understanding of traumatic growth in the face of terrorism: Moving from meaning cognitions to doing what is meaningful. *Applied Psychology*, 56(3), 345-366.

Holland, P. W. (1986). Statistics and causal inference. *Journal of the American Statistical Association*, 81 (396), 945-960.

Horowitz, M. J. (1976). *Stress response syndromes*. Northvale: Aronson.

Horowitz, M. J. (1980). *Psychological response to serious life events*. In: Hamilton, V., Warburton, D. (Eds.), Human Stress and Cognition. New York: Wiley.

Horowitz, M. J. (1982). *Stress response syndromes and their treatment*. In: Goldberger, L., Breznitz, S. (Eds.), Handbook of Stress. New York: Free Press.

Horowitz, M. J. (1983). *Psychological response to serious life events*. In: Breznitz, S. (Ed.), The Denial of Stress. New York: International Universities Press.

Ickovics, J. R., Meade, C. S., Kershaw, T. S., Milan, S., Lewis, J. B., & Ethier, K. A. (2006). Urban teens: Trauma, posttraumatic growth, and emotional distress among female adolescents. *Journal of Consulting and Clinical Psychology*, 74(5), 841-850.

Ingram, R. E. (1990). Self-focused attention in clinical disorders: review and a conceptual model. *Psychological bulletin*, 107(2), 156-176.

Ionio, C., Mascheronia, E., & Blasioa, P. D. (2018). The centrality of events scale for Italian adolescents: integrating traumatic experience into one's identity and its relation to posttraumatic stress disorder symptomatology. *Europe's journal of psychology*, 14(2), 359-372.

Ivarsson, T., Granqvist, P., Gillberg, C., & Broberg, A. G. (2010). Attachment states of mind in adolescents with Obsessive-Compulsive Disorder and/or depressive disorders: a controlled study. *European child & adolescent psychiatry*, 19(11), 845-853.

Janet, P. (1901). *The Mental State of the Hysterics: A study of mental stigmata and mental accidents*. GP Putnam's sons.

Janoff-Bulman, R. (1989). Assumptive worlds and the stress of traumatic events: Applications of the schema construct. *Social cognition*, 7(2), 113-136.

Janoff-Bulman, R. (1992). *Shattered Assumptions: Towards a New Psychology of Trauma*. New York, NY: Free Press.

Jardin, C., Venta, A., Newlin, E., Ibarra, S., & Sharp, C. (2017). Secure attachment moderates the relation of sexual trauma with trauma symptoms among adolescents from an inpatient psychiatric facility. *Journal of Interpersonal Violence*, 32(10), 1565-1585.

Jayawickreme, N., Jayawickreme, E., & Foa, E. B. (2013). Using the individualism-collectivism construct to understand cultural differences in PTSD. In K. Gow & M. Celinski (Eds.), *Mass trauma: Impact and recovery issues* (pp. 55-76). Nova Science Publishers.

Ji, K., & Finkelhor, D. (2015). A meta-analysis of child physical abuse prevalence in China. *Child Abuse & Neglect*, 43, 61-72.

Jin, Y. , Deng, H. , An, J. , & Xu, J. (2019). The prevalence of PTSD symptoms and depressive symptoms and related predictors in children and adolescents 3 years after the Ya'an earthquake. *Child Psychiatry & Human Development*, 50(2), 300-307.

Johnson, H. , & Thompson, A. (2008). The development and maintenance of posttraumatic stress disorder (PTSD) in civilian adult survivors of war trauma and torture: A review. *Clinical Psychology Review*, 28, 36-47.

Jones, P. J. (2017). *Networktools: Tools for identifying important nodes in networks*. R package version 1. 1. 0. https://CRAN.R-project.org/package=networktools

Jones, P. J. , Heeren, A. , & McNally, R. J. (2017a). Commentary: A network theory of mental disorders. *Frontiers in Psychology*, 8, 1305.

Jones, P. J. , Ma, R. , & McNally, R. J. (2019). Bridge centrality: A network approach to understanding co-morbidity. Manuscript submitted for publication. *Multivariate Behavioral Research*, 56(2), 353-367.

Joseph, S. (2012). *What doesn't kill us: a guide to overcoming adversity and moving forward*. UK: Hachette.

Joseph, S. , & Linley, P. A. (2004). Positive therapy: A positive psychological theory of therapeutic practice. In P. A. Linley & S. Joseph (Eds.), *Positive psychology in practice* (pp. 354-368). John Wiley & Sons, Inc. .

Joubert, D. , Webster, L. , & Hackett, R. K. (2012). Unresolved attachment status and trauma-related symptomatology in maltreated adolescents: An examination of cognitive mediators. *Child psychiatry & human development*, 43(3), 471-483.

Kabat-Zinn, J. (1994). *Wherever you go, there you are: Mindfulness meditation in everyday life*. UK: Hachette.

Kaczkurkin, A. N. , Zang, Y. , Gay, N. G. , Peterson, A. L. , Yarvis, J. S. ,

Borah, E. V., ... & STRONG STAR Consortium. (2017). Cognitive emotion regulation strategies associated with the DSM-5 posttraumatic stress disorder criteria. *Journal of traumatic stress*, 30(4), 343-350.

Kaplow, J. B., Gipson, P. Y., Horwitz, A. G., Burch, B. N., & King, C. A. (2014). Emotional suppression mediates the relation between adverse life events and adolescent suicide: Implications for prevention. *Prevention science*, 15, 177-185.

Keane, T. M., Brief, D. J., Pratt, E. M., & Miller, M. W. (2007). Assessment of PTSD and its comorbidities in adults. In: Friedman, M. J., Keane, T. M., Resick, P. A. (Eds.), *Handbook of PTSD* (pp. 279-305). New York: The Guilford Press.

Keller, T. E., Salazar, A. M., & Courtney, M. E. (2010). Prevalence and timing of diagnosable mental health, alcohol, and substance use problems among older adolescents in the child welfare system. *Children and youth services review*, 32(4), 626-634

Kilmer, R. P., & Gil-Rivas, V. (2010). Exploring posttraumatic growth in children impacted by Hurricane Katrina: Correlates of the phenomenon and developmental considerations. *Child Development*, 81, 1211-1227.

Kilmer, R. P., Gil-Rivas, V., Tedeschi, R. G., Cann, A., Calhoun, L. G., & Buchanan, T., et al. (2009). Use of the revised posttraumatic growth inventory for children (PTGI-C-R). *Journal of traumatic stress*, 22(3), 248-253.

Kilpatrick, D. G., Acierno, R., Resnick, H. S., Saunders, B. E., & Best, C. L. (1997). A 2-year longitudinal analysis of the relationships between violent assault and substance use in women. *Journal of Consulting and Clinical Psychology*, 65(5), 834-847.

King, L. A., Scollon, C. K., Ramsey, C., & Williams, T. (2000). Stories of life transition: Subjective well-being and ego development in parents of

children with Down Syndrome. *Journal of Research in Personality*, 34
(4), 509-536.

Koster, E. H. , De Lissnyder, E. , Derakshan, N. , & De Raedt, R. (2011).
Understanding depressive rumination from a cognitive science
perspective: the impaired disengagement hypothesis. *Clinical
psychology review*, 31(1), 138-145.

Krueger, R. F. , Markon, K. E. , Patrick, C. J. , & Iacono, W. G. (2005).
Externalizing psychopathology in adulthood: A dimensional-spectrum
conceptualization and its implications for DSM-V. *Journal of Abnormal
Psychology*, 114(4), 537-550.

La, G. A. , Silverman, W. K. , Vernberg, E. M. , & Prinstein, M. J. (1996).
Symptoms of posttraumatic stress in children after Hurricane Andrew:
a prospective study. *Journal of Consulting and Clinical Psychology*,
64, 712-723

Lahav, Y. , Solomon, Z. , & Levin, Y. (2016). Posttraumatic growth and
perceived health: The role of posttraumatic stress symptoms. *American
Journal of Orthopsychiatry*, 86(6), 693.

Lampe, A. (2002). The prevalence of childhood sexual abuse, physical abuse
and emotional neglect in Europe. *Zeitschrift fur Psychosomatische
Medizin und Psychotherapie*, 48(4), 370-380.

Lancaster, S. L. , Klein, K. R. , Nadia, C. , Szabo, L. , & Mogerman, B.
(2015). An integrated model of posttraumatic stress and growth.
Journal of Trauma & Dissociation, 16(4), 399-418.

Landolt, M. A. , Schnyder, U. , Maier, T. , Schoenbucher, V. , & Mohler-
Kuo, M. (2013). Trauma exposure and posttraumatic stress disorder in
adolescents: A national survey in Switzerland. *Journal of Traumatic
Stress*, 26(2), 209-216.

LaRocca, M. A. , & Avery, T. J. (2020). Combat experiences link with posttraumatic growth among veterans across conflicts: The influence of ptsd and depression. *The Journal of nervous and mental disease*, 208 (6),445-451.

Laub Huizenga, L. A. (2011). *Expressive Writing Intervention for Teens Whose Parents Have Cancer*. Doctoral dissertation, University of Kansas.

Laufer, A. , Hamama-Raz, Y. , Levine, S. Z. , & Solomon, Z. (2009). Posttraumatic growth in adolescence: The role of religiosity, distress, and forgiveness. *Journal of Social and Clinical Psychology*, 28(7), 862-880.

Laufer, A. , & Solomon, Z. (2006). Posttraumatic symptoms and posttraumatic growth among Israeli youth exposed to terror incidents. *Journal of Social and Clinical Psychology*, 25(4),429-447.

Lauritzen, S. L. (1996). *Graphical models*. Gloucestershire, England: Clarendon Press.

Lee, W. K. (2016). Psychological characteristics of self-harming behavior in Korean adolescents. *Asian journal of psychiatry*, 23,119-124.

Lepore, S. J. , & Greenberg, M. A. (2002). Mending broken hearts: Effects of expressive writing on mood, cognitive processing, social adjustment and health following a relationship breakup. *Psychology and Health*, 17 (5),547-560.

Levine, S. Z. , Laufer, A. , Hamama-Raz, Y. , Stein, E. , & Solomon, Z. (2008). Posttraumatic growth in adolescence: examining its components and relationship with PTSD. *Journal of traumatic stress*, 21 (5), 492-496.

Levine, S. Z. , Laufer, A. , Stein, E. , Hamama-Raz, Y. , & Solomon, Z. (2009). Examining the relationship between resilience and posttraumatic growth. *Journal of Traumatic Stress: Official*

Publication of The International Society for Traumatic Stress Studies, 22(4), 282-286.

Li, X. , Wang, Z. , Hou, Y. , Wang, Y. , Liu, J. , & Wang, C. (2014). Effects of childhood trauma on personality in a sample of Chinese adolescents. *Child abuse & neglect*, 38(4), 788-796.

Li, Y. , Xu, Y. , & Chen, Z. (2015). Effects of the behavioral inhibition system (BIS), behavioral activation system (BAS), and emotion regulation on depression: A one-year follow-up study in Chinese adolescents. *Psychiatry research*, 230(2), 287-293.

Lin, D. , Li, X. , Fan, X. , & Fang, X. (2011). Child sexual abuse and its relationship with health risk behaviors among rural children and adolescents in Hunan, China. *Child abuse & neglect*, 35(9), 680-687.

Linley, P. A. , & Joseph, S. (2004). Positive change following trauma and adversity: A review. *Journal of traumatic stress: official publication of the international society for traumatic stress studies*, 17(1), 11-21.

Liotti, G. (1992). Disorganized/disoriented attachment in the etiology of the dissociative disorders. *Dissociation*, 5, 196-204.

Liotti, G. (1994). Disorganized attachment and dissociative experiences: An illustration of the developmental-ethological approach to cognitive therapy. In K. T. Kuehlwein & H. Rosen (Eds.), *Cognitive therapies in action: Evolving innovative practice. The Jossey Bass social and behavioral science series* (pp. 213-239). San Francisco, CA: Jossey-Bass.

Liu, L. , Wang, L. , Cao, C. , Qing, Y. , & Armour, C. (2016). Testing the dimensional structure of DSM-5 posttraumatic stress disorder symptoms in a nonclinical trauma exposed adolescent sample. *Journal of child psychology and psychiatry, and allied disciplines*, 57(2), 204-212.

London, M. J. , Lilly, M. M. , & Pittman, L. (2015). Attachment as a mediator between community violence and posttraumatic stress symptoms among adolescents with a history of maltreatment. *Child Abuse & Neglect*, 42, 1-9.

Lu, D. , Wang, W. , Qiu, X. , Qing, Z. , Lin, X. , Liu, F. , ... & Liu, X. (2020). The prevalence of confirmed childhood trauma and its' impact on psychotic-like experiences in a sample of Chinese adolescents. *Psychiatry research*, 287, 112897.

Lubke, G. , & Muthén, B. O. (2007). Performance of factor mixture models as a function of model size, covariate effects, and class-specific parameters. *Structural Equation Modeling*, 14(1), 26-47.

Lyons-Ruth, K. , Dutra, L. , Schuder, M. R. , & Bianchi, I. (2006). From infant attachment disorganization to adult dissociation: Relational adaptations or traumatic experiences? *Psychiatric Clinics of North America*, 29(1), 63-86.

Ma, X. , Liu, X. , Hu, X. , Qiu, C. , Wang, Y. , Huang, Y. , ... & Li, T. (2011). Risk indicators for post-traumatic stress disorder in adolescents exposed to the 5. 12 Wenchuan earthquake in China. *Psychiatry research*, 189(3), 385-391.

MacDonald, H. Z. , Beeghly, M. , Grant-Knight, W. , Augustyn, M. , Woods, R. W. , Cabral, H. , et al. (2008). Longitudinal association between infant disorganized attachment and childhood posttraumatic stress symptoms. *Development & Psychopathology*, 20(2), 493-508.

MacLeod, C. , Rutherford, E. , Campbell, L. , Ebsworthy, G. , & Holker, L. (2002). Selective attention and emotional vulnerability: Assessing the causal basis of their association through the experimental manipulation of attentional bias. *Journal of Abnormal Psychology*, 111(1), 107-123.

Madjar, N. , Segal, N. , Eger, G. , & Shoval, G. (2019). Exploring particular facets of cognitive emotion regulation and their relationships with nonsuicidal self-injury among adolescents. *Crisis*,40(4),280-286.

Maercker, A. , & Zoellner, T. (2004). The Janus face of self-perceived growth: toward a two-component model of posttraumatic growth. *Psychological Inquiry*,15(1),41-48.

Main,M. , & Hesse, E. (1990). Parents' unresolved traumatic experiences are related to infant disorganized attachment status: Is frightened and/ or frightening parental behavior the linking mechanism? In M. T. Greenberg,D. Cicchetti, & E. M. Cummings (Eds.), *Attachment in the preschool years: Theory, research, and intervention* (pp. 161-182). Chicago: University of Chicago Press.

Marcia,J. E. (1994). Identity and Psychotherapy. In S. L. Archer (Ed.), *Interventions for adolescent identity development* (pp. 29-46). Sage Publications, Inc.

Marsee, M. A. (2008). Reactive aggression and posttraumatic stress in adolescents affected by hurricane Katrina. *Journal of Clinical Child & Adolescent Psychology*,37(3),519-529.

Marshall, R. D. , Olfson, M. , Hellman, F. , Blanco, C. , Guardino, M. , & Struening, E. L. (2001). Comorbidity, impairment, and suicidality in subthreshold PTSD. *The American Journal of Psychiatry*,158(9), 1467-1473.

Martin, L. L. , & Clore, G. L. (2001). *Theories of mood and cognition: A user's guidebook*. Mahwah, NJ: Erlbaum.

Marusak,H. A. , Martin, K. R. , Etkin, A. , & Thomason, M. E. (2015). Childhood trauma exposure disrupts the automatic regulation of emotional processing. *Neuropsychopharmacology*,40(5),1250-1258.

Masten, A. S. (2014). Global perspectives on resilience in children and youth. *Child development*,85(1),6-20.

Mathews, A. , & MacLeod, C. (2005). Cognitive vulnerability to emotional disorders. *Annual review of clinical psychology*, 1, 167-195.

Mazor, Y. , Gelkopf, M. , Mueser, K. T. , & Roe, D. (2016). Posttraumatic growth in psychosis. *Frontiers in Psychiatry*, 7, 202.

McChesney, G. C. , Adamson, G. , & Shevlin, Mark. (2015). A latent class analysis of trauma based on a nationally representative sample of US adolescents. *Social psychiatry and psychiatric epidemiology*, 50(8), 1207-1217.

Menon, V. , Shanmuganathan, B. , Thamizh, J. S. , Arun, A. B. , Kuppili, P. P. , & Sarkar, S. (2018). Personality traits such as neuroticism and disability predict psychological distress in medically unexplained symptoms: A three-year experience from a single center. *Personality and mental health*, 12(2), 145-154.

McDonald, R. P. , & Ho, M. H. (2002). Principles and practice in reporting structural equation analyses. *Psychological methods*, 7(1), 64-82.

McLaughlin, K. A. , Koenen, K. C. , Hill, E. D. , Petukhova, M. , Sampson, N. A. , Zaslavsky, A. M. , & Kessler, R. C. (2013). Trauma exposure and posttraumatic stress disorder in a national sample of adolescents. *Journal of the American Academy of Child & Adolescent Psychiatry*, 52(8), 815-830.

McMillen, C. , Zuravin, S. , & Rideout, G. (1995). Perceived benefit from child sexual abuse. *Journal of consulting and clinical psychology*, 63(6), 1037-1043.

McMillen, J. C. , Zima, B. T. , Scott, L. D. , Jr, Auslander, W. F. , Munson, M. R. , Ollie, M. T. , & Spitznagel, E. L. (2005). Prevalence of psychiatric disorders among older youths in the foster care system. *Journal of the American Academy of Child & Adolescent Psychiatry*, 44(1), 88-95.

McNally, R. J. (2017). Networks and nosology in posttraumatic stress disorder. *JAMA Psychiatry*, 74(2), 124-125.

McNally, R. J. , Robinaugh, D. J. , Wu, G. W. , Wang, L. , Deserno, M. K. , & Borsboom, D. (2015). Mental disorders as causal systems a network approach to posttraumatic stress disorder. *Clinical Psychological Science*, 3(6), 836-849.

Meesters, C. , Merckelbach, H. , Muris, P. , & Wessel, I. (2000). Autobiographical memory and trauma in adolescents. *Journal of Behavior Therapy and Experimental Psychiatry*, 31(1), 29-39.

Merikangas, K. R. , He, J. P. , Burstein, M. , Swanson, S. A. , Avenevoli, S. , Cui, L. , ... & Swendsen, J. (2010). Lifetime prevalence of mental disorders in US adolescents: results from the National Comorbidity Survey Replication-Adolescent Supplement (NCS-A). *Journal of the American Academy of Child & Adolescent Psychiatry*, 49 (10), 980-989.

Meyerson, D. A. , Grant, K. E. , Carter, J. S. , & Kilmer, R. P. (2011). Posttraumatic growth among children and adolescents: A systematic review. *Clinical psychology review*, 31(6), 949-964.

Mikulincer, M. , Gillath, O. , & Shaver, P. R. (2002). Activation of the attachment system in adulthood: Threat-related primes increase the accessibility of mental representations of attachment figures. *Journal of Personality and Social Psychology*, 83(4), 881-895.

Mikulincer, M. , & Shaver, P. R. (2003). The attachment behavioral system in adulthood: Activation, psychodynamics, and interpersonal processes. In M. P. Zanna (Ed.), *Advances in experimental social psychology* (Vol. 35, pp. 53-152). San Diego, CA: Academic Press.

Mikulincer, M. , & Shaver, P. R. (2007). Boosting attachment security to promote mental health, prosocial values, and inter-group tolerance. *Psychological Inquiry*, 18(3), 139-156.

Mikulincer, M. , Shaver, P. R. , & Solomon, Z. (2015). An attachment perspective on traumatic and posttraumatic reactions. In M. P. Safir, H. S. Wallach, & A. " S. " Rizzo (Eds.), *Future directions in post-traumatic stress disorder* (pp. 79-96). Boston, MA: Springer.

Milam, J. E. , Ritt-Olson, A. , & Unger, J. B. (2004). Posttraumatic growth among adolescents. *Journal of Adolescent Research*, 19(2), 192-204.

Miller, M. W. , Greif, J. L. , & Smith, A. A. (2003). Multidimensional personality questionnaire profiles of veterans with traumatic combat exposure: Internalizing and externalizing subtypes. *Psychological Assessment*, 15(2), 205-215.

Miller, M. W. , Kaloupek, D. G. , Dillon, A. L. , & Keane, T. M. (2004). Externalizing and internalizing subtypes of combat related PTSD: a replication and extension using the PSY-5 scales. *Journal of abnormal psychology*, 113(4), 636-645.

Mitchell, K. S. , Mazzeo, S. E. , Schlesinger, M. R. , Brewerton, T. D. , & Smith, B. N. (2012). Comorbidity of partial and subthreshold PTSD among men and women with eating disorders in the national comorbidity survey-replication study. *International Journal of Eating Disorders*, 45(3), 307-315.

Mostafaei, S. , Kabir, K. , Kazemnejad, A. , Feizi, A. , Mansourian, M. , Keshteli, A. H. ,... & Ghadirian, F. (2019). Explanation of somatic symptoms by mental health and personality traits: application of Bayesian regularized quantile regression in a large population study. *BMC psychiatry*, 19(1), 1-8.

Motreff, Y. , Baubet, T. , Pirard, P. , Rabet, G. , Petitclerc, M. , Stene, L. E. ,... & Vandentorren, S. (2020). Factors associated with PTSD and partial PTSD among first responders following the Paris terror attacks in November 2015. *Journal of psychiatric research*, 121, 143-150.

Murad, K. , & Thabet, A. A. (2017). The relationship between traumatic experience, posttraumatic stress disorder, resilience, and posttraumatic growth among adolescents in Gaza strip. *Glob. J. Intellect. Dev. Disabil.* , 555616.

Murphy, S. , Hansen, M. , Elklit, A. , Chen, Y. Y. , Ghazali, S. R. , & Shevlin, M. (2018). Alternative models of DSM-5 PTSD: examining diagnostic implications. *Psychiatry research* , 262, 378-383.

Ndetei, D. M. , Ongecha-Owuor, F. A. , Khasakhala, L. , Mutiso, V. , Odhiambo, G. , & Kokonya, D. A. (2007). Traumatic experiences of Kenyan secondary school students. *Journal of child and adolescent mental health* , 19(2), 147, 155.

Neimeyer, R. A. (2006). Complicated grief and the quest for meaning: A constructivist contribution. *OMEGA-Journal of Death and Dying* , 52 (1), 37-52.

Nelson, S. D. (2011). The posttraumatic growth path: An emerging model for prevention and treatment of trauma-related behavioral health conditions. *Journal of Psychotherapy Integration* , 21(1), 1-42.

Nerken, I. R. (1993). Grief and the reflective self: Toward a clearer model of loss resolution and growth. *Death Studies* , 17(1), 1-26.

Newman, M. E. J. , & Girvan, M. (2004). Finding and evaluating community structure in networks. *Physical Review* , 69(2 Pt 2), 26113.

Nijdam, M. J. , Baas, M. A. , Olff, M. , & Gersons, B. P. (2013). Hotspots in trauma memories and their relationship to successful trauma-focused psychotherapy: A pilot study. *Journal of Traumatic Stress* , 26 (1), 38-44.

Nishikawa, S. , Fujisawa, T. X. , Kojima, M. , & Tomoda, A. (2018). Type and timing of negative life events are associated with adolescent Depression. *Frontiers in Psychiatry* , 9, 41.

Nolen-Hoeksema, S. (1991). Responses to depression and their effects on the duration of depressive episodes. *Journal of Abnormal Psychology*, 100 (4), 569-582.

Nye, E. C., Katzman, J., Bell, J. B., Kilpatrick, J., Brainard, M., & Haaland, K. Y. (2008). Attachment organization in Vietnam combat veterans with posttraumatic stress disorder. *Attachment & Human Development*, 10(1), 41-57.

Nylund, K. L., Asparouhov, T., & Muthén, B. O. (2007). Deciding on the number of classes in latent class analysis and growth mixture modeling: A Monte Carlo simulation study. *Structural Equation Modeling*, 14 (4), 535-569.

O'Leary, V. E., & Ickovics, J. R. (1995). Resilience and thriving in response to challenge: an opportunity for a paradigm shift in women's health. *Women's health (Hillsdale, NJ)*, 1(2), 121-142.

Owens, M., Goodyer, I. M., Wilkinson, P., Bhardwaj, A., Abbott, R., & Croudace T et al. (2012). 5-HTTLPR and early childhood adversities moderate cognitive and emotional processing in adolescence. *PLoS ONE*, 7(11), e48482.

Oyserman, D., & Lee, S. W. (2008). Does culture influence what and how we think? Effects of priming individualism and collectivism. *Psychological bulletin*, 134(2), 311-342.

Parent, M. C. (2013). Handling item-level missing data: Simpler is just as good. *The Counseling Psychologist*, 41(4), 568-600.

Park, C. L., Cohen, L. H., & Murch, R. L. (1996). Assessment and prediction of stress-related growth. *Journal of personality*, 64 (1), 71-105.

Pat-Horenczyk, R., Kenan, A. M., Achituv, M., & Bachar, E. (2014). Protective factors based model for screening for posttraumatic distress in adolescents. *Child & Youth Care Forum*, 43(3), 339-351.

Pearlman, L. A. , & Saakvitne, K. W. (1995). *Trauma and the therapist: Countertransference and vicarious traumatization in psychotherapy with incest survivors*. New York, US: W. W. Norton & Company.

Pennebaker, J. W. (1993). Putting stress into words: Health, linguistic, and therapeutic implications. *Behaviour Research and Therapy*, 31 (6), 539-548.

Perkonigg, A. , Pfister, H. , Stein, M. B. , Höfler, M. , Lieb, R. , Maercker, A. , & Wittchen, H. U. (2005). Longitudinal course of posttraumatic stress disorder and posttraumatic stress disorder symptoms in a community sample of adolescents and young adults. *The American Journal of Psychiatry*, 162(7), 1320-1327.

Perrotta, G. (2019). Psychological trauma: definition, clinical contexts, neural correlations and therapeutic approaches recent discoveries. *Current Research in Psychiatry and Brain Disorders*, CRPBD-100006.

Pietrzak, R. H. , Goldstein, R. B. , Southwick, S. M. , & Grant, B. F. (2011). Prevalence and Axis I comorbidity of full and partial posttraumatic stress disorder in the United States: Results from Wave 2 of the National Epidemiologic Survey on Alcohol and Related Conditions. *Journal of Anxiety Disorders*, 25(3), 456-465.

Pillemer, D. B. (2003). Directive functions or autobiographical memory: the guiding power of the specific episode. *Memory (Hove, England)*, 11 (2), 193-202.

Plener, P. L. , Singer, H. , & Goldbeck, L. (2011). Traumatic events and suicidality in a German adolescent community sample. *Journal of Traumatic Stress*, 24(1), 121-124.

Proffitt, D. , Cann, A. , Calhoun, L. G. , & Tedeschi, R. G. (2007). Judeo-Christian clergy and personal crisis: Religion, posttraumatic growth and well being. *Journal of Religion and Health*, 46(2), 219-231.

Quan, L. , Zhen, R. , Yao, B. , Zhou, X. , & Yu, D. (2017). The role of perceived severity of disaster, rumination, and trait resilience in the relationship between rainstorm-related experiences and PTSD amongst Chinese adolescents following rainstorm disasters. *Archives of psychiatric nursing*, 31(5), 507-515.

Regier, D. A. , Kuhl, E. A. , & Kupfer, D. J. (2013). The DSM-5: Classification and criteria changes. *World Psychiatry*, 12(2), 92-98.

Rey Peña, L. , & Extremera Pacheco, N. (2012). Physical-verbal aggression and depression in adolescents: The role of cognitive emotion regulation strategies. *Universitas Psychologica*, 11(4), 1245-1254.

Riggs, S. A. , Paulson, A. , Tunnell, E. , Sahl, G. , Atkinson, H. , & Ross, C. A. (2007). Attachment, personality, and psychopathology among adult inpatients: Self-reported romantic attachment style versus Adult Attachment Interview states of mind. *Development and Psychopathology*, 19(1), 263-291.

Robinaugh, D. J. , & McNally, R. J. (2011). Trauma centrality and PTSD symptom severity in adult survivors of childhood sexual abuse. *Journal of traumatic stress*, 24(4), 483-486.

Robinaugh, D. J. , & McNally, R. J. (2013). Remembering the past and envisioning the future in bereaved adults with and without complicated grief. *Clinical Psychological Science*, 1(3), 290-300.

Robinaugh, D. J. , Millner, A. J. , & McNally, R. J. (2016). Identifying highly influential nodes in the complicated grief network. *Journal of Abnormal Psychology*, 125(6), 747-757.

Rucklidge, J. J. (2006). Psychosocial functioning of adolescents with and without pediatric bipolar disorder. *Journal of Affective Disorders*, 91 (2-3), 181-188.

Russell, J. M. , Koran, L. M. , Rush, J. , Hirschfeld, R. M. , Harrison, W. , Friedman, E. S. , ... & Keller, M. (2001). Effect of concurrent anxiety on response to sertraline and imipramine in patients with chronic depression. *Depression and Anxiety*, 13(1), 18-27.

Russell, J. D. , Neill, E. L. , Carrio n, V. G. , & Weems, C. F. (2017). The network structure of posttraumatic stress symptoms in children and adolescents exposed to disasters. *Journal of the American Academy of Child and Adolescent Psychiatry*, 56(8), 669-677.

Ryff, C. D. , & Singer, B. (1998). The role of purpose in life and personal growth in positive human health. In P. T. P. Wong & P. S. Fry (Eds.), *The human quest for meaning : A handbook of psychological research and clinical applications* (pp. 213-235). Mahwah, NJ: Lawrence Erlbaum Associates, Inc.

Sadler-Gerhardt, C. , Reynolds, C. , Britton, P. , & Kruse, S. (2010). Women breast cancer survivors: Stories of change and meaning. *Journal of Mental Health Counseling*, 32(3), 265-282.

Salazar, A. M. , Keller, T. E. , Gowen, L. K. , & Courtney, M. E. (2013). Trauma exposure and PTSD among older adolescents in foster care. *Social psychiatry and psychiatric epidemiology*, 48(4), 545-551.

Sar, V. , & Ozturk, E. (2006). What is trauma and dissociation? *Journal of Trauma Practice*, 4(1-2), 7-20.

Scheeringa, M. S. , & Zeanah, C. H. (2008). Reconsideration of harm's way: Onsets and comorbidity patterns of disorders in preschool children and their caregivers following Hurricane Katrina. *Journal of Clinical Child and Adolescent Psychology*, 37(3), 508-518.

Sayar, K. , Kose, S. , Grabe, H. J. , & Topbas, M. (2005). Alexithymia and dissociative tendencies in an adolescent sample from Eastern Turkey. *Psychiatry and Clinical Neurosciences*, 59(2), 127-134.

Scales, P. C. , Benson, P. L. , Leffert, N. , & Blyth, D. A. (2000). Contribution of developmental assets to the prediction of thriving among adolescents. *Applied Developmental Science*, 4(1), 27-46.

Schimmenti, A. , & Caretti, V. (2016). Linking the overwhelming with the unbearable: developmental trauma, dissociation, and the disconnected self. *Psychoanalytic Psychology*, 33(1), 106-128.

Schuettler, D. , & Boals, A. (2011). The path to posttraumatic growth versus posttraumatic stress disorder: contributions of event centrality and coping. *Journal of Loss and Trauma*, 16(2), 180-194.

Seth, P. , Jackson, J. M. , DiClemente, R. J. , & Fasula, A. M. (2017). Community trauma as a predictor of sexual risk, marijuana use, and psychosocial outcomes among detained African American female adolescents. *Vulnerable Children and Youth Studies*, 12(4), 353-359.

Setliff, A. E. , & Marmurek, H. H. (2002). The mood regulatory function of autobiographical recall is moderated by self-esteem. *Personality and Individual Differences*, 32(4), 761-771.

Silva, R. R. , Alpert, M. , Munoz, D. M. , Singh, S. , Matzner, F. , & Dummit, S. (2000). Stress and vulnerability to posttraumatic stress disorder in children and adolescents. *The American Journal of Psychiatry*, 157(8), 1229-1235.

Simpson, J. A. , & Rholes, W. S. (2002). Fearful-avoidance, disorganization, and multiple working models: Some directions for future theory and research. *Attachment & Human Development*, 4(2), 223-229.

Slanbekova, G. K. , Chung, M. C. , Ayupova, G. T. , Kabakova, M. P. , Kalymbetova, E. K. , & Korotkova-Ryckewaert, N. V. (2019). The relationship between posttraumatic stress disorder, interpersonal sensitivity and specific distress symptoms: the role of cognitive emotion regulation. *Psychiatric Quarterly*, 90(4), 803-814.

Snyder,C. R. (2002). Hope theory: Rainbows in the mind. *Psychological Inquiry*,13(4),249-275.

Solomon,E. P. , & Heide,K. M. (1999). Type Ⅲ trauma: Toward a more effective conceptualization of psychological trauma. *International Journal of Offender Therapy and Comparative Criminology*,43(2), 202-210.

Steel, C. (2016). Cognitive emotion regulation as a mediator between posttraumatic stress symptoms and hypomanic personality within a non-clinical population. *Behavioral and cognitive psychotherapy*, 44 (1),104-111.

Stikkelbroek,Y. ,Bodden,D. H. ,Kleinjan,M. ,Reijnders,M. , & van Baar, A. L. (2016). Adolescent depression and negative life events, the mediating role of cognitive emotion regulation. *PloS one*, 11 (8),e0161062.

Stovall-McClough, K. C. , & Cloitre, M. (2006). Unresolved attachment, PTSD, and dissociation in women with childhood abuse histories. *Journal of consulting and clinical psychology*,74(2),219-228.

Sun,J. (2012). *Educational stress among Chinese adolescents : Measurement, risk factors and associations with mental health*. Doctoral dissertation, Queensland University of Technology.

Sun,J. ,Dunne,M. P. ,Hou,X. Y. , & Xu,A. Q. (2011). Educational stress scale for adolescents: development,validity,and reliability with Chinese students. *Journal of Psychoeducational Assessment*,19(6),534-546.

Svedin, C. G. , Nilsson, D. , & Lindell, Charlotta. (2004). Traumatic experiences and dissociative symptoms among Swedish adolescents. A pilot study using Dis-Q-Sweden. *Nordic Journal of Psychiatry*,58(5), 349-355.

Szentágotai-Tătar, A. , & Miu, A. C. (2016). Individual differences in emotion regulation, childhood trauma and proneness to shame and guilt in adolescence. *PLoS One*, 11(11), e0167299.

Taku, K. , Cann, A. , Calhoun, L. G. , & Tedeschi, R. G. (2008). The factor structure of the Posttraumatic Growth Inventory: A comparison of five models using confirmatory factor analysis. *Journal of Traumatic Stress*, 21(2), 158-164.

Taku, K. , Cann, A. , Tedeschi, R. G. , & Calhoun, L. G. (2017). Psychoeducational intervention program about posttraumatic growth for Japanese high school students. *Journal of loss and trauma*, 22(4), 271-282.

Taku, K. , Tedeschi, R. G. , Shakespeare-Finch, J. , Krosch, D. , David, G. , Kehl, D. , ... & Calhoun, L. G. (2021). Posttraumatic growth (PTG) and posttraumatic depreciation (PTD) across ten countries: Global validation of the PTG-PTD theoretical model. *Personality and Individual Differences*, 169, 110222.

Taylor, S. E. , & Armor, D. A. (1996). Positive illusions and coping with adversity. *Journal of personality*, 64(4), 873-898.

Taylor, S. E. , & Brown, J. D. (1988). Illusion and well-being: a social psychological perspective on mental health. *Psychological bulletin*, 103 (2), 193-210.

Tedeschi, R. G. , & Calhoun, L. G. (1995). *Trauma and transformation: Growing in the aftermath of suffering*. Thousand Oaks, CA: Sage.

Tedeschi, R. G. , & Calhoun, L. G. (1996). The posttraumatic growth inventory: Measuring the positive legacy of trauma. *Journal of Traumatic Stress*, 9(3), 455-471.

Tedeschi, R. G. , & Calhoun, L. G. (2004). Posttraumatic growth: conceptual foundations and empirical evidence. *Psychological Inquiry*, 15 (1), 1-18.

Tedeschi, R. , Calhoun, L. , & Cann, A. (2007). Evaluating resource gain: Understanding and misunderstanding posttraumatic growth. *Applied Psychology: An International Review*, 56, 396-406.

Tedeschi, R. G. , & Kilmer, R. P. (2005). Assessing strengths, resilience, and growth to guide clinical interventions. *Professional Psychology: Research and Practice*, 36(3), 230-237.

Tedeschi, R. G. , Park, C. L. , & Calhoun, L. G. (Eds.). (1998). *Posttraumatic growth: Positive changes in the aftermath of crisis*. New York: Routledge.

Tedeschi, R. G. , Shakespeare-Finch, J. , Taku, K. , & Calhoun, L. G. (2018). *Posttraumatic growth: Theory, research, and applications*. New York: Routledge.

Tennen, H. , Affleck, G. , Urrows, S. , Higgins, P. , & Mendola, R. (1992). Perceiving control, construing benefits, and daily processes in rheumatoid arthritis. *Canadian Journal of Behavioural Science/Revue canadienne des sciences du comportement*, 24(2), 186-203.

Terr, L. C. (1991). Childhood traumas: An outline and overview. *American Journal of Psychiatry*, 148(1), 10-20.

Thomas, E. A. , Hamrick, L. A. , Owens, G. P. , & Tekie, Y. T. (2019). Posttraumatic growth among undergraduates: Contributions from adaptive cognitive emotion regulation and emotional intelligence. *Traumatology*, 26(1), 68-73.

Thompson, R. A. (1991). Emotional regulation and emotional development. *Educational Psychology Review*, 3, 269-307.

Thomson, P. , & Jaque, S. V. (2018). Depersonalization, adversity, emotionality, and coping with stressful situations. *Journal of Trauma & Dissociation*, 19(2), 143-161.

Tian, Y. X. , Wu, X. C. , Wang, W. C. , & Zhou, X. (2018). The relation between attachment and PTSD/PTG among adolescents after the Wenchuan earthquake: the mediating roles of cognitive reappraisal and expressive suppression [Chinese]. *Psychological Development and Education*, 34(1), 105-111.

Tian, Y. X. , Zhou, X. , Wu, X. C. , & Zeng, M. (2016). The moderating role of emotion regulation between PTSD and PTG. *Chinese Journal of Clinical Psychology*, 24(3), 480-483.

Torres, S. A. , & DeCarlo Santiago, C. (2017). Culture and educational stress and internalizing symptoms among Latino adolescents: the role of ethnic identity. *Journal of Educational and Psychological Consultation*, 27 (3), 344-366.

Triplett, K. N. , Tedeschi, R. G. , Cann, A. , Calhoun, L. G. , & Reeve, C. L. (2012). Posttraumatic growth, meaning in life, and life satisfaction in response to trauma. *Psychological Trauma: Theory, Research, Practice, and Policy*, 4(4), 400-410.

Turton, P. , Hughes, P. , Fonagy, P. , & Fainman, D. (2004). An investigation into the possible overlap between PTSD and unresolved responses following stillbirth: An absence of linkage with only unresolved status predicts infant disorganization. *Attachment & Human Development*, 6(3), 241-261.

Vagos, P. , da Silva, D. R. , Brazão, N. , & Rijo, D. (2018). The Centrality of Events Scale in Portuguese adolescents: validity evidence based on internal structure and on relations to other variables. *Assessment*, 25 (4), 527-538.

van der Kolk, B. A. (2005). Developmental trauma disorder: Towards a rational diagnosis for chronically traumatized children. *Psychiatric Annals*, 35(5), 401-408.

van der Kolk, B. A. , & Fisler, R. (1995). Dissociation and the fragmentary nature of traumatic memories: overview and exploratory study. *Journal of Traumatic Stress*, 8(4), 505-525.

van Hoof, M. J. , van Lang, N. D. , Speekenbrink, S. , van IJzendoorn, M. H. , & Vermeiren, R. R. (2015). Adult Attachment Interview differentiates adolescents with Childhood Sexual Abuse from those with clinical depression and non-clinical controls. *Attachment & Human Development*, 17(4), 354-375.

Van Loey, N. E. , Klein-König, I. , De Jong, A. E. E. , Hofland, H. W. C. , Vandermeulen, E. , & Engelhard, I. M. (2018). Catastrophizing, pain and traumatic stress symptoms following burns: A prospective study. *European journal of pain*, 22(6), 1151-1159.

Vishnevsky, T. , Cann, A. , Calhoun, L. G. , Tedeschi, R. G. , & Demakis, G. J. (2010). Gender differences in self-reported posttraumatic growth: A meta-analysis. *Psychology of Women Quarterly*, 34(1), 110-120.

Vloet, A. , Simons, M. , Vloet, T. D. , Sander, M. , Herpertz-Dahlmann, B. , & Konrad, K. (2014). Long-term symptoms and posttraumatic growth in traumatized adolescents: findings from a specialized outpatient clinic. *Journal of traumatic stress*, 27(5), 622-625.

Vogt, D. , King, D. , & King, L. (2007). Risk pathways in PTSD: making sense of the literature. In Friedman, M. , Kean, T. , Resick, P. (Eds.), *Handbook of PTSD: Science and Practice* (pp. 99-116). New York: Guildford.

Walburg, V. , Zakari, S. , & Chabrol, H. (2014). Role of academic burnout in suicidal ideas among adolescent. *Neuropsychiatrie de l'Enfance et de l'Adolescence*, 62(1), 28-32.

Wamser-Nanney, R. , Howell, K. H. , & Schwartz, L. E. (2018). The moderating role of trauma type on the relationship between event centrality of the traumatic experience and mental health outcomes. *Psychological trauma: theory, research, practice and policy*, 10(5), 499-507.

Wang, N., Chung, M. C., & Wang, Y. (2020). The relationship between posttraumatic stress disorder, trauma centrality, posttraumatic growth and psychiatric co-morbidity among Chinese adolescents. *Asian journal of psychiatry*, 49, 101940.

Wang, N., Chung, M. C., Liu, F., & Wang, Y. (2022). Posttraumatic stress on Chinese adolescents' posttraumatic growth: The role of trauma centrality and emotion regulation. *Current Psychology*, 42, 20015-20027.

Wang, Y., & Chung, M. C. (2020). Linking rejection sensitivity, shyness and unsociability with posttraumatic stress disorder and psychiatric co-morbidity among Chinese adolescents. *Psychiatric Quarterly*, 91(2), 309-319.

Wang, Y., Chung, M. C., & Wang, N. (2021). Parenting revisited: Profiles and associations with psychological distress among traumatized Chinese adolescents. *Current Psychology*, 42, 1-10.

Wang, X., Yang, L., Gao, L., Yang, J., Lei, L., & Wang, C. (2017). Childhood maltreatment and Chinese adolescents' bullying and defending: The mediating role of moral disengagement. *Child abuse & neglect*, 69, 134-144.

Watkins, E. R. (2008). Constructive and unconstructive repetitive thought. *Psychological Bulletin*, 134(2), 163-206.

Waugh, C. E., Fredrickson, B. L., & Taylor, S. F. (2008). Adapting to life's slings and arrows: Individual differences in resilience when recovering from an anticipated threat. *Journal of Research in Personality*, 42(4), 1031-1046.

Waugh, A. , Kiemle, G. , & Slade, P. (2018). What aspects of posttraumatic growth are experienced by bereaved parents? A systematic review. *European journal of psychotraumatology* , 9(1) , 1506230.

Waysman, M. , Schwarzwald, J. , & Solomon, Z. (2001). Hardiness: An examination of its relationship with positive and negative long-term changes following trauma. *Journal of Traumatic Stress : Official Publication of the International Society for Traumatic Stress Studies* , 14(3) , 531-548.

Weathers, F. W. , Litz, B. T. , Keane, T. M. , Palmieri, P. A. , Marx, B. P. , & Schnurr, P. P. (2013). *The PTSD Checklist for DSM*-5 (*PCL*-5). https://www.ptsd.va.gov

Weiss, D. S. , Marmar, C. R. , Schlenger, W. E. , Fairbank, J. A. , Jordan, B. K. , Hough, R. L. , & Kulka, R. A. (1992). The prevalence of lifetime and partial post-traumatic stress disorder in Vietnam theater veterans. *Journal of Traumatic Stress* , 5 , 365-376.

Wen, Z. L. , Hau, K. T. , & Marsh, H. W. (2004). Structural equation model testing: cutoff criteria for goodness of fit indices and Chi-square test. *Acta Psychologica Sinica* , 36 , 186-194.

West, M. , Rose, S. , Spreng, S. , & Adam, K. (2000). The Adolescent Unresolved Attachment Questionnaire: The assessment of perceptions of parental abdication of caregiving behavior. *The Journal of Genetic Psychology* , 161(4) , 493-503.

Wilson, J. (2006). The posttraumatic self. In Wilson, J. (Ed.), *The Posttraumatic Self : Restoring Meaning and Wholeness to Personality*. New York: Routledge.

Wolfe, D. A. , Scott, K. , Wekerle, C. , & Pittman, Anna-Lee. (2001). Child maltreatment: Risk of adjustment problems and dating violence in adolescence. *Journal of the American Academy of Child and*

Adolescent Psychiatry, 40(3), 282-289.

Wright, M. O. D. , Masten, A. S. , & Narayan, A. J. (2013). Resilience processes in development: Four waves of research on positive adaptation in the context of adversity. In Goldstein, S. , Brooks, R. (eds), *Handbook of Resilience in Children* (pp. 15-37). Boston, MA: Springer.

Wu, X. C. , Wang, W. C. , Zhou X. , Chen, Q. Y. , & Lin, C. D. (2018). Investigation on mental health state of adolescents after 8. 5 years of Wenchuan earthquake [Chinese]. *Psychological Development and Education*, 34(1), 80-89.

Wu, X. C. , Zhou X. , Chen, J. L. , & Zeng, M. (2015). The relationship among deliberate rumination, posttraumatic stress disorder and posttraumatic growth: Evidence from longitudinal study of adolescents after Wenchuan earthquake [Chinese]. *Psychological Development and Education*, 31(3), 334-341.

Wu, X. , Zhang, Y. , Lin, C. , & Zang, W. (2013). The effect of disaster exposure on PTSD of primary and secondary students: Mediating and moderating effects. *Psychological Development and Education*, 29(6), 641-648.

Xiao, Y. , Jiang, L. , Yang, R. , Ran, H. , Wang, T. , He, X. , . . . & Lu, J. (2021). Childhood maltreatment with school bullying behaviors in Chinese adolescents: A cross-sectional study. *Journal of affective disorders*, 281, 941-948.

Xu, W. , Ding, X. , Goh, P. H. , & An, Y. (2018). Dispositional mindfulness moderates the relationship between depression and posttraumatic growth in Chinese adolescents following a tornado. *Personality and Individual Differences*, 127, 15-21.

Xu, W. , Fu, G. , An, Y. , Yuan, G. , Ding, X. , & Zhou, Y. (2018).

Mindfulness, posttraumatic stress symptoms, depression, and social functioning impairment in Chinese adolescents following a tornado: mediation of posttraumatic cognitive change. *Psychiatry research*, 259, 345-349.

Xu, W. , Jiang, H. , Zhou, Y. , Zhou, L. , & Fu, H. (2019). Intrusive rumination, deliberate rumination, and posttraumatic growth among adolescents after a tornado: the role of social support. *The Journal of Nervous and Mental Disease*, 207(3), 152-156.

Yalom, I. D. , & Lieberman, M. A. (1991). Bereavement and heightened existential awareness. *Psychiatry*, 54(4), 334-345.

Yan, Y. W. , Lin, R. M. , Su, Y. K. , & Liu, M. Y. (2018). The relationship between adolescent academic stress and sleep quality: a multiple mediation model. *Social Behavior and Personality: An International Journal*, 46(1), 63-78.

Yang, H. , Wang, L. , Cao, C. , Cao, X. , Fang, R. , Zhang, J. , & Elhai, J. D. (2017). The underlying dimensions of DSM-5 PTSD symptoms and their relations with anxiety and depression in a sample of adolescents exposed to an explosion accident. *European journal of psychotraumatology*, 8(1), 1272789.

Ying, L. , Chen, C. , Lin, C. , Greenberger, E. , Wu, X. , & Jiang, L. (2015). The relationship between posttraumatic stress symptoms and suicide ideation among child survivors following the Wenchuan earthquake. *Suicide and Life-threatening Behavior*, 45(2), 230-242.

Ying L, Wang Y, Lin C, Chen C (2016) Trait resilience moderated the relationships be- tween PTG and adolescent academic burnout in a post-disaster context. *Personality and Individual Differences*, 90, 108-112.

Ying, L. , Wu, X. , Lin, C. , & Jiang, L. (2014). Traumatic severity and trait resilience as predictors of posttraumatic stress disorder and depressive symptoms among adolescent survivors of the Wenchuan earthquake. *PloS one*, 9(2), 89401.

Yu, X. N., Lau, J. T. F., Zhang, J. X., Mak, W. W. S., Choi, K. C., Lui, W. W. S., & Chan, E. Y. Y. (2010). Posttraumatic growth and reduced suicidal ideation among adolescents at month 1 after the Sichuan Earthquake. *Journal of affective disorders*, 123(1-3), 327-331.

Yu, G., Li, S., & Zhao, F. (2020). Childhood maltreatment and prosocial behavior among Chinese adolescents: Roles of empathy and gratitude. *Child abuse & neglect*, 101, 104319.

Yuan, G. Z., Xu, W., Liu, Z., & An, Y. Y. (2018). Resilience, posttraumatic stress symptoms, and posttraumatic growth in Chinese adolescents after a tornado: the role of mediation through perceived social support. *The Journal of nervous and mental disease*, 206(2), 130-135.

Zakari, S., Walburg, V., & Chabrol, H. (2008). Study of burnout, depression and suicidal thoughts among French high-school students. *Journal de Thérapie Comportementale et Cognitive*, 18(3), 113-118.

Zatzick, D. F., Grossman, D. C., Russo, J., Pynoos, R., Berliner, L., Jurkovich, G., ... & Rivara, F. P. (2006). Predicting posttraumatic stress symptoms longitudinally in a representative sample of hospitalized injured adolescents. *Journal of the American Academy of Child & Adolescent Psychiatry*, 45(10), 1188-1195.

Zeller, M. H., Noll, J. G., Sarwer, D. B., Reiter-Purtill, J., Rofey, D. L., Baughcum, A. E., Peugh, J., Courcoulas, A. P., Michalsky, M. P., Jenkins, T. M., & Becnel, J. N. (2015). Child maltreatment and the adolescent patient with severe obesity: Implications for clinical care. *Journal of Pediatric Psychology*, 40(7), 640-648.

Zerach, G. (2015). Secondary growth among former prisoners of war's adult children: the result of exposure to stress, secondary traumatization, or personality traits. *Psychological trauma :theory,research,practice and policy*,7(4),313-323.

Zhao, X. F. , Zhang, Y. L. , & Li, L. F. (2004). Childhood abuse: An investigation of 435 middle school students. *Chinese Journal of Clinical Psychology*,12,377-379.

Zhou,X. ,& Wu,X. (2016). Understanding the roles of gratitude and social support in posttraumatic growth among adolescents after Ya'an earthquake: A longitudinal study. *Personality and Individual Differences*,101,4-8.

Zhou,X. ,Wu,X. ,An,Y. ,& Chen,J. (2014). The roles of rumination and social support in the associations between core belief challenge and post-traumatic growth among adolescent survivors after the Wenchuan earthquake [Chinese]. *Acta Psychologica Sinica*,46,1509-1520.

Zhou,X. ,Wu,X. C. , & Chen,J. L. (2015). Moderating effect of resilience between PTSD and posttraumatic growth. *Chinese Journal of Clinical Psychology*,23(3),512-516.

Zhou,X. , Wu, X. C. , Zeng, M. , & Tian, Y. X. (2016). The relationship between emotion regulation and PTSD/PTG among adolescents after the Ya' an earthquake: the moderating role of social support. *Acta Psychologica Sinica*,48(8),969-980.

Zhou, X. , Wu, X. , & Zhen, R. (2017). Understanding the relationship between social support and posttraumatic stress disorder/posttraumatic growth among adolescents after Ya'an earthquake: The role of emotion regulation. *Psychological Trauma: Theory, Research, Practice, and Policy*,9(2),214-221.

Zhou,X. ,Wu,X. C. , & Zhen,R. (2018). Self-esteem and hope mediate the relations between social support and posttraumatic stress disorder and growth in adolescents following the Ya'an earthquake. *Anxiety,Stress, & Coping*,31(1),32-45.

Zlotnick, C., Franklin, C. L., & Zimmerman, M. (2002). Does " subthreshold " posttraumatic stress disorder have any clinical relevance? *Comprehensive Psychiatry*, 43(6), 413-419.

Zoellner, T., & Maercker, A. (2006). Posttraumatic growth in clinical psychology—a critical review and introduction of a two-component model. *Clinical psychology review*, 26(5), 626-653.